ADDITIONAL ADVANCE PRAISE FOR
WHAT IF I HAVE A C-SECTION?

"The current rise in the popularity of caesarean delivery demands an unbiased and informed look at the risks and benefits of this major surgical procedure. *What If I Have a C-Section?* provides exactly that. It's must reading for all pregnant women."

—Christiane Northrup, M.D., author of *Women's Bodies, Women's Wisdom* (Bantam, 1998) and *The Wisdom of Menopause* (Bantam, 2001)

"Ms. Rubin has given all expectant mothers a wonderful shower gift—a practical, concise, yet comprehensive book on Cesarean delivery. Since one in four American women will delivery their babies via this route, many unexpectedly—it is a good book to have handy. Ms. Rubin covers the common reasons for C-sections, ways to minimize your risk, how the procedure is performed and what the recovery is like. She also covers the controversy surrounding trials of labor after prior C-sections. Having observed firsthand her journalistic skill, objectivity and thoroughness in covering women's health issues, I am not at all surprised by the excellence of this book."

—Charles J. Lockwood, M.D., chair, Department of Obstetrics, Gynecology and Reproductive Sciences, Yale University School of Medicine

"This book is a wonderful, reassuring resource for mothers-to-be everywhere. I highly recommend it."

—Helain J. Landy, M.D., director, Maternal-Fetal Medicine Fellowship Program, and director, Labor and Delivery, Georgetown University Hospital

WHAT IF I HAVE
A C-SECTION?

How to Prepare • How to Decide
• How to Recover Quickly

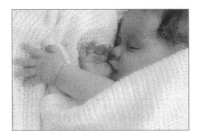

RITA RUBIN, *USA Today* medical reporter
Foreword by Mark B. Landon, M.D., vice-chair of the department
of obstetrics and gynecology, The Ohio State University

RODALE

© 2004 by Rita Rubin

All rights reserved. No part of this publication may be reproduced or transmitted in any form or by any means, electronic or mechanical, including photocopying, recording, or any other information storage and retrieval system, without the written permission of the publisher.

Printed in the United States of America
Rodale Inc. makes every effort to use acid-free ♾, recycled paper ♻.

Book design by Christina Gaugler
Cover/interior photograph © Dia Max/Getty Images

Library of Congress Cataloging-in-Publication Data

Rubin, Rita.
    What if I have a C-section? / Rita Rubin ; foreword by Mark B. Landon.
       p.   cm.
    Includes bibliographical references and index.
    ISBN 1–57954–907–1 paperback
    1. Cesarean section—Popular works. I. Title.
    RG761.R83   2004
    618.8'6—dc22   2004010461

Distributed to the trade by Holtzbrinck Publishers

2 4 6 8 10 9 7 5 3 1 paperback

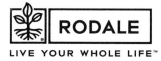

RODALE

LIVE YOUR WHOLE LIFE™

FOR MORE OF OUR PRODUCTS
WWW.RODALESTORE.COM
(800) 848-4735

In loving memory of my parents, Herman Rubin, M.D. and Audrey Miriam Dobkin Rubin and, with much love, for Mike, Hannah, and Aliza

CONTENTS

FOREWORD

Cesarean childbirth remains one of the most controversial issues in obstetrics and is of great interest to women, health care providers, and institutions. As cesarean section rates have skyrocketed in the United States, many pregnant women have come to expect the strong possibility of unplanned cesarean birth; yet others, perhaps less informed, participate in childbirth education with limited focus on the preparation for potential cesarean delivery.

What If I Have a C-Section? is a magnificent resource for primigravid (first time pregnant) women as well as those having undergone cesarean delivery. This guide covers virtually every major topic relevant to cesarean birth and offers the reader good advice, while dispelling myths concerning methods which might reduce the chance of unnecessary cesarean section. Women who have experienced cesarean section and VBAC vividly recall their stories and give unique perspectives to the data and information cited in this marvelous monograph. Rita Rubin has done a remarkably artful job assimilating and interpreting in clear terms much of the voluminous scientific data concerning cesarean section. She frames the important questions, provides answers when possible, and points out gaps in our knowledge just as well. This is particularly true in her discussion of VBAC and of "cesarean section on demand," a practice which is likely to increase in the future.

This book also contains practical advice about pain control, breastfeeding, and recovery for women scheduled for or recently post-cesarean delivery. The controversies surrounding cesarean childbirth are numerous and the debate will likely continue in the medical community, and elsewhere for years to come. Pregnant women must seek information about cesarean section and become partners with their health care providers in planning for childbirth. *What If I Have a C-Section?* provides much of the groundwork in preparing women for an open discussion on this subject.

—Mark B. Landon, M.D.,
professor and vice-chair, department of obstetrics and gynecology,
The Ohio State University College of Medicine and Public Health;
chief of clinical obstetrics, The Ohio State University Hospitals,
Columbus, Ohio

ACKNOWLEDGMENTS

First, I'd like to thank all the women who so generously shared their enlightening and sometimes entertaining perspectives on birthing babies. Your wisdom and your wit shaped this book. In addition, I'd like to express my gratitude to the physicians and researchers who graciously took the time to answer my questions: Zane Brown, M.D., Gunhilde Buchsbaum, M.D., Deborah Cohan, M.D., G. Willy Davila, M.D., Eugene Declerq, Ph.D., Bruce Flamm, M.D., Roger Freeman, M.D., Fredric Frigoletto, M.D., Roger Goldberg, M.D., Mary Hannah, M.D., W. Benson Harer Jr., M.D., Erlend Hem, M.D., Jay Iams, M.D., K.S. Joseph, M.D., Helain Landy, M.D., Russell Laros, M.D., Michele Lauria, M.D., Lawrence Leeman, M.D., Elliot Levine, M.D., Charles Lockwood, M.D., Mona Lydon-Rochelle, Ph.D., C.N.M., George Macones, M.D., Antonio Alberto Nogueira, M.D., Maureen Porter, M.D., Laura Riley, M.D., Guri Rortveit, M.D., Kathleen Rice Simpson, PhD., R.N., Gordon Smith, M.D., Catherine Spong, M.D., Javier Vizoso, M.D., David Walters, M.D., Carolyn Zelop, M.D., and Jun Zhang, Ph.D.

I'd especially like to thank Mark Landon, M.D., for his insight into C-sections in particular and maternity care in general.

Gregory Phillips at the American College of Obstetricians and Gynecologists and Robert Bock at the National Institute for Child

Health and Human Development were a great help in connecting me with the experts.

I am indebted to my agent (and fellow former Poppy preschool parent) Djana Pearson Morris for her encouragement and guidance, and to my editor at Rodale, Mariska van Aalst, for patiently helping me make the transition from daily journalist to book author.

Thanks also to my editors at *USA Today*, Susan Weiss, Linda Kauss, and Glenn O'Neal, for their support.

My sister, Ronna Rubin, scoured Nashville for women with great tales to tell about C-sections, and for that I am grateful.

Most of all, I'd like to thank my wonderful husband, Michael Broder—computer maven, dad extraordinaire and all-around great guy—and our delightful daughters, Hannah and Aliza Broder, for putting up with me during a year of lost weekends and late nights spent working on this book.

INTRODUCTION

Congratulations. If you're reading these words, you're most likely a mom-to-be looking forward to the big day when you'll finally meet your baby. Or if you're not pregnant yet, you're seriously considering it. You think you know what to expect in labor and delivery. After all, your friends and relatives have regaled you with their birth stories and shown off their cuddly newborns' first photos. But what you might not realize is that you have a greater than 1-in-4 chance of delivering your baby via major abdominal surgery, otherwise known as a C-section.

The U.S. C-section rate is now the highest it's ever been. In fact, for a complex variety of reasons, cesareans have become one of the most commonly performed medical procedures in the United States and other developed countries.

But most women who end up having a C-section weren't planning to. They thought they were going to deliver vaginally and never considered otherwise—until, perhaps, after hours of contractions and pushing. Generally, lessons learned from weeks of childbirth classes are of little help in understanding a cesarean delivery. In fact, childbirth courses often seem aimed at convincing women that anything short of a drug-free "natural" delivery constitutes failure.

Not surprisingly, one of the biggest complaints from women who end up having cesareans is that they felt vastly unprepared.

After an induction and nearly 24 hours of labor, Andrea, now 39, delivered her 3½-year-old daughter via C-section. Cesarean deliveries merited maybe a half-hour of discussion in her childbirth course. Looking back, Andrea says, she recognizes that, like many, her childbirth courses focused on a wholistic, natural approach. It presented epidurals and C-sections as something to be avoided at all costs. Although she never missed a class, Andrea says, "I wasn't prepared to have a C-section in any sense."

Susan M., 29, read just about every book she could find about pregnancy and childbirth when pregnant with her daughter 3 years ago. She felt as ready as she could be, and she looked forward to a relatively uneventful birth. But nothing prepared her for preeclampsia—a serious pregnancy-related condition that causes blood pressure to soar—and the resulting emergency C-section under general anesthesia. "The advice I would give any mother-to-be is to make sure you educate yourself about childbirth, including cesarean section delivery," says Susan, who also delivered her second daughter by C-section. "I wish I knew more about preeclampsia before I was pregnant. I wish I knew more about cesarean sections before I was pregnant."

Jaime, now 26, delivered both of her daughters, ages 3 and 1, by unplanned C-sections. Afterward, she didn't feel as well as she'd expected. Once she got home from the hospital, she searched in vain for information about recovering from cesareans. "Maybe what I was going through was normal, maybe it wasn't. I can't put into words what it was like during my recovery time," she says now. She couldn't find anything to reassure her that it was perfectly normal to feel pain in her middle even after she left the hospital. After all, a C-section is major abdominal surgery. "I thought, 'Wait a minute, something's not right here,'" she recalls. "Of course, there are a lot of Web sites about giving birth naturally."

As Andrea, Susan M. and Jaime discovered, you can't be certain about having a vaginal delivery until your newborn is actually nestled in your arms. If you're pregnant—or even if you're just considering pregnancy—this book can help you prepare for that uncharted territory called childbirth. Each chapter focuses on the latest research into the risks and benefits of C-sections and of vaginal births after C-sections, or VBACs. Whether you want to avoid having a C-section or are considering asking for one upfront, this book will help you sort out the medicine from the myth. You'll explore the fascinating origins of the operation we now call cesarean section (one tidbit: Julius Caesar probably had little to do with it) and why it has become so common in the United States and other western countries. You'll learn the main reasons cesareans are performed and steps you can take to enhance your chances of delivering vaginally, whether or not you've had a prior C-section. You'll read about the growing trend of "patient-choice" C-sections among women concerned about the long-term health consequences of a vaginal delivery. In addition, you'll get detailed information about the operation itself—what's really going on behind that surgical drape. And you'll get tips about how best to speed your recovery.

Throughout the book, you'll find tales of real-life birth experiences, ranging from women who would never consider delivering vaginally to those who searched long and hard to find a doctor and hospital who would let them. In each chapter, "Talking Points" lay out issues to discuss with your doctor or midwife, while "Words from the Wise" features good advice from women who've been there and from medical experts. At the end of the book, you'll find a list of resources that can further help you prepare for delivery, whether it ends up being a vaginal birth or a cesarean.

Knowledge really is power. If you end up having a C-section, your surgery and recovery can go more smoothly when you know what to expect. If you hope to avoid a C-section, it's important to know what factors increase your chances of having one. Some are avoidable, such as an obstetrician who has a high cesarean delivery rate, while others—such as a breech baby who cannot be turned—are not.

What you won't find on these pages is a discourse on the one "right" way to give birth, because there is no such thing. The right way to give birth is any way that minimizes the risk of harm to you and your baby. For most women, that means an uncomplicated vaginal delivery accomplished without the help of forceps or vacuum extraction. For others, the right way to give birth could be a vaginal delivery with forceps or vacuum extraction, a preplanned C-section before their first contraction, or a cesarean after hours of labor. And for a small minority of women, the right way to give birth is by emergency cesarean under general anesthesia.

Sometimes, the right way to deliver doesn't become clear until afterward; and, at least initially, it may not jibe with your notions of the ideal delivery. At first, Andrea says, her unplanned C-section "did make me feel that I had failed somehow as a woman. On the other hand, what I wanted most was a healthy child. You defer to expert advice."

Kathryn's first three children were delivered by unplanned C-sections. "I had this one friend who kept saying, 'You're really missing out, you're really missing out,'" says Kathryn, 41. "I was determined to have a vaginal birth." With the help of a remarkably supportive obstetrician, she had four vaginal deliveries, followed by two planned cesareans. With the benefit of all of these experiences, she wants women to know: "Either way you deliver, you're not missing out on anything."

Like Kathryn, Cheryl's birth experiences pretty much covered the gamut. She delivered her first two sons, now ages 16 and 14, by C-sections, the second under general anesthesia because the epidural wasn't working and there wasn't time to correct it. After her eldest was born, she remembers feeling blue. "I was actually depressed that second or third day. I was kind of crying and everything," she says. "Stupidly, I felt I wouldn't be a real woman unless I delivered naturally." Cheryl, 43, got her wish and had successful VBACs with sons three and four, now ages 11 and 8. She came to realize that how you deliver has nothing to do with your worth as a woman. "It was a ridiculous opinion, but I don't think I could know that. I think the bottom line is having a healthy baby. If it turns out that you need a C-section, it's certainly not a failure, and it's silly to think of it that way. Just be happy that you have a healthy baby."

After reading this book, you might end up changing your mind about C-sections, you might not. In any case, you shouldn't be wracked with guilt if your plans for a low-tech birth go awry or if you decide from the outset that you want a cesarean. No matter how you deliver, familiarizing yourself with the range of options can help you relax during labor (if you labor at all) and delivery and speed your recovery, so you can delight in the real point of it all: your healthy, happy baby.

PART I

THE COMPLETE C-SECTION GUIDE

CHAPTER I

WILL I HAVE A C-SECTION?

A look at some of the common medical reasons for C-Sections

Annie, 35, took a Lamaze class to prepare for the birth of her first child, now 6 months old. She doesn't remember learning anything about C-sections, but maybe that's because she, like most pregnant women, never expected to have one. "I was so focused on the fact that I was going to have a natural childbirth and on strategies for dealing with that: breathing exercises, stretching."

But when she arrived at the hospital to be induced, her doctor discovered that her son wasn't head-down in her uterus—the optimal position for delivery. He was in the breech position, and these days, few doctors are willing to deliver a breech baby vaginally. "My doctor really danced around it for a minute," Annie recalls. " I think he was very afraid of my reaction."

Her doctor explained that it might be possible for him to turn the baby head-down for a vaginal delivery, but the thought made her squeamish—so she resigned herself to having a cesarean. "It was not a hard decision, but I was a little bit bummed at first. I looked at giving birth as sort of a challenge. When they told me it was going to be a C-section, they were kind of taking that away from me."

Annie quickly got used to the idea that she was not going to deliver vaginally. "I was very proud that I was relaxed about the entire thing. I figured people have had babies for years. All of my friends have had babies. It's going to be a life-altering experience. The worst thing I could do was to make myself a nervous wreck."

Annie is part of a growing trend in the United States, and chances are higher than ever that you will be, too. Cesarean delivery is the most common major surgical procedure among U.S. women of reproductive age. In fact, it's one of the most common major surgical procedures in the United States, period.

In 2002, 261 out of every 1,000 babies born in the United States were delivered by C-section—the highest rate ever, although not nearly as high as in Brazil and some other Latin American countries. If the trend continues, half of all U.S. babies could be delivered by cesarean by the time your grandchildren are born (if not sooner). Some observers think cesareans have already become too common—that perhaps as many as half of them are unnecessary. The World Health Organization, for example, says that no more than 150 out of every 1,000 babies should be delivered by C-section. Others think that trying to reduce the number of cesareans is unnecessary, if not foolhardy. "Setting a target rate is an authoritarian approach to healthcare delivery," Harvard OB/GYNs Fredric Frigoletto and Benjamin Sachs wrote in 1999 in *The New England*

Looking Back

Abdominal deliveries are mentioned in ancient Hindu, Egyptian, Greek, and Roman folklore and in the Talmud. In fact, Greek mythology provides several examples of gods from Zeus onward delivering babies through their mothers' bellies.

Journal of Medicine. "It implies that women should have no say in their own care."

Although experts aren't sure what the optimal cesarean delivery rate is, they know it shouldn't be zero. Clearly, C-sections can preserve the health of mothers and babies and sometimes even save their lives. Doctors are virtually in agreement that certain situations require a cesarean delivery, although these cases represent only a small proportion of all C-sections. If you're diagnosed with any of the following, you can pretty much count on having a C-section:

- *Breech presentation.* A baby who, like Annie's son, isn't head-down in your pelvis
- *Cephalopelvic disproportion.* A baby whose head is deemed to big to fit through your pelvis
- *Placenta previa.* A baby whose exit through the birth canal is blocked by the placenta

But you'll be happy to know that these three conditions aren't very common. Only about three or four out of every 100 babies isn't head-down at the time of delivery. True cephalopelvic disproportion happens mainly in the rare woman who is not just petite, but has an abnormally small pelvis—perhaps because of an injury suffered in an automobile accident. And placenta previa occurs in only about one out of every 200 births.

Other reasons for planned cesareans include severe high blood pressure, herpes, and multiple babies; but research suggests that most women with these conditions deliver vaginally. Now you're beginning to enter the wide gray zone of C-section land. They don't call medicine an art for nothing. In the majority of cases, you could present two doctors with the same pregnant woman, and one might recommend a cesarean while the other holds out for a vaginal delivery. And a third doctor might have a tough time deciding who's right.

Sometimes, medical judgment isn't the only factor at play here. Some doctors (as well as many of their patients) perceive cesareans to be less risky than vaginal deliveries for babies and mothers. They believe that if you have a C-section, you'll be less likely to sue them for malpractice. OB/GYNs are among the specialists most likely to get sued, according to malpractice insurance industry data, so you can't blame them for practicing defensive medicine.

It's those gray-area cases that account for the most dramatic variations in C-section rates among doctors and hospitals. You can see these variations even among doctors practicing at the same hospital, as well as at different hospitals in the same city. For example, in Pennsylvania hospitals, the 1999 rates for women considered at low risk for a C-section—basically, first-time moms whose babies were full-term and head-down—ranged from about 8½ percent to 28 percent. In other words, if you'd delivered in 1999 at the Pennsylvania hospital with the highest cesarean rate rather than the lowest (and there's no reason to think the situation was any different in other states), you would have more than tripled your chance of having a C-section. If you don't have an obvious reason for a planned cesarean, such as a baby who's lying sideways, is there any way to predict you're going to end up with one anyway? Unfortunately, no, although researchers are hunting for clues. Most C-sections are still performed after hours of labor. But researchers at the University of Colorado Health Sciences Center recently uncovered five possible signs of a likely C-section that your doctor can assess within the first couple of hours after you're admitted to the hospital in labor:

- Preeclampsia (also called toxemia)
- How much your cervix dilates in those first 2 hours
- Your weight

- How far along you are in your pregnancy
- How far down your baby is in your pelvis

If you and another woman were nearly the same as far as the other four factors, but you had preeclampsia and she didn't, you'd be nearly six times more likely than she would to have a C-section. If you and this hypothetical other woman were the same except that she didn't dilate as much as you did during those first 2 hours in the hospital, she'd be four times more likely to have a cesarean. And if you were the same except for the fact that you weighed 25 pounds more than she did, you'd be 1½ times more likely to wind up in the O.R.

Now, this was only one study—and a retrospective one at that (in other words, it looked at women who had already delivered). The challenge will be to see if the five clues really can predict the chance of a C-section in laboring women. If so, doctors someday might be able to use them to help patients decide whether they should continue aiming for a vaginal delivery.

MIDLIFE MOTHERHOOD:
WHAT'S AGE GOT TO DO WITH IT?

If you're trying to figure out your chances of having a C-section, look in your wallet. If you have a health insurance card, research shows that you're more likely to deliver by cesarean than a woman who's uninsured or covered by Medicaid, the state/federal program for low-income Americans. And your driver's license yields more information than all those diplomas hanging in your obstetrician's office—that is, if you were honest about your age and weight when you applied for your license!

If you were over your ideal weight before you conceived, or you gained more than 40 pounds while pregnant, you're more likely to deliver by cesarean. Those extra pounds raise your risk of developing diabetes or high blood pressure, which in turn increases your chance of having a C-section. Even if you avoid those complications, it's important to remember that the more weight you gain, the bigger your baby might be—and bigger babies tend to be harder to push out. Studies by researchers at the National Institutes of Health and elsewhere also suggest that the heavier you are, the longer your labor might be.

And even if you're a rail, simply being closer to your 40th than your 30th birthday raises your chance of delivering by cesarean, especially if it's your first baby. If you're one of those so-called "mature" pregnant women (don't you love those terms?) preparing to deliver your first baby, you're in good company. Growing numbers of women who delayed childbearing because of graduate school, career advancement, infertility, or late and second marriages are now tossing hair dye along with diapers into their shopping carts. Just look at these numbers from the National Center for Health Statistics, part of the federal Centers for Disease Control and Prevention:

- In 2002, birth rates for women age 35 to 39 and age 40 to 44 were the highest in more than 30 years—41 births per 1,000 women and 8 per 1,000 women, respectively.
- From 1990 to 2002, the number of babies born to women age 40 to 44 nearly doubled—from 48,607 to 95,788.
- The birth rate for women age 45 to 49 has been stable since 2000, but the actual number of births to women in this age group more than quadrupled between 1984 and 2002. That's because there are more of these women—thanks to the baby boomer bulge—and they're more likely to give birth, partly because of infertility treatments.

The majority of pregnant women over 35, or even over 40, deliver healthy babies. But there's no getting around the fact that the older you are, the more likely you are to deliver your baby by C-section. For example, Harvard researchers found that 43 percent of first-time mothers age 40 and older who delivered at Boston's Brigham and Women's Hospital in 1998 had cesareans, compared to only 12 percent of those under 35. One reason for that disparity is pretty simple: The older you get, the more likely you are to experience pregnancy complications that predispose you to a cesarean. They include:

- Multiples (often a result of infertility treatments)
- Breech babies
- Illnesses such as diabetes and high blood pressure

But even if you don't have any of the above risk factors, you should be aware that simply being a first-time mother who's at least 35 years old increases your chance of having a C-section. Part of that may be physiological; part of it may be cultural. A San Francisco study of 8,500 first-time moms who delivered full-term, head-down babies found that the older they were, the longer they labored. Their cervixes dilated more slowly, and it took longer for them to push their babies out. Not surprisingly, then, the older they were, the more likely they were to receive oxytocin (frequently referred to by one of its brand names, Pitocin) to ramp up their labor. But it's not like your uterus suddenly heads south when you hit 35. Here's a cheery thought: The study found that the chance that your uterus has lost its oomph actually begins to increase when you're in your early 20s—long before you begin to entertain thoughts of Botox or bifocals.

Even if you're as healthy as a horse and your uterus is chugging along just fine, your age might still mean the difference between a C-section and a vaginal delivery. Perhaps you've spent many years and many thousands of dollars in your quest for

motherhood. It's understandable that you—and your doctor—
might be a little more anxious about your baby's safety than if
you were 10 or 15 years younger. This condition has been
dubbed "precious baby" or "premium baby" syndrome, and it
can lead to a lower threshold for performing C-sections. In other
words, if there's even the slightest suggestion that your baby is in
trouble during labor, your doctor would resort to a cesarean faster
than with a younger patient who could easily get pregnant again.
You might find this line of thinking perfectly logical, or you
might not. But however you feel about it, you should discuss
your feelings with your doctor well in advance of your due date.
No matter what your age, remember that you're not destined to
have your labor stall or your doctor choose a C-section without
your knowledge or consent.

FEET (OR BOTTOM) FIRST:
WHEN BABY IS BREECH

Babies in the womb have better moves than any contortionist you'd
see at the circus. In their first 36 weeks, they take advantage of their
relatively roomy quarters and change position frequently. Three or

TALKING POINT

If you're expecting your first child at age 35 or older,
ask your doctor whether he might be quicker to perform a C-section on you than on a younger patient,
all other factors being equal.

four weeks before they're due to exit, though, they usually settle into a head-down position. By that time, space is getting pretty tight, so they're unlikely to change position.

But about three or four babies out of every 100 prefer not to be upside down, making a vaginal delivery tricky, although not necessarily impossible. Most doctors have become leery of delivering breech babies vaginally, due to liability concerns, so vaginal delivery of these babies is rapidly becoming a lost art. In 2001, 86 percent of their moms gave birth via C-section.

Sometimes babies' buttocks are the lowest part of their body, with their legs extended straight up in front of them (talk about contortionists!). This is called a frank breech presentation, and it's the main position (other than head-down) that some doctors are willing to deliver vaginally. Sometimes babies are sitting cross-legged, although their buttocks are still the lowest part of their body. This is called a complete breech, and vaginal delivery is still possible. Sometimes babies' knees or feet are closest to the birth canal, a position called footling breech, which virtually always requires delivery by C-section. And sometimes babies are sideways, the transverse lie position, which requires a cesarean.

There's a reason babies are normally born head-first. Think about it: The head is by far the biggest part of baby's body. It stretches mom's cervix, allowing the rest of his body to slide through fairly easily. If his feet or rear end come out first, it gets more difficult to guide the baby's head out. In addition, there's a higher risk of the umbilical cord slipping through the cervix and into the birth canal before the baby exits—a serious condition called a prolapsed cord. This can stop the flow of blood through the cord. Several factors further increase the risk of complications in breech babies delivered vaginally:

- Older mother
- Footling breech position
- Estimated birth weight of less than 5½ pounds or more than 8¾ pounds
- Prolonged labor
- Doctor inexperienced in delivering breech babies vaginally

Just because your baby is head-up or sideways doesn't mean there are other problems. It's often hard to explain why a baby isn't head-down, or in the vertex position. Breech babies are more common in women who have been pregnant before, are carrying more than one baby, or have placenta previa. Babies are also more likely to be breech if mom's uterus is shaped abnormally or contains too much or too little amniotic fluid or if there are abnormal growths, such as fibroids. And preemies are more likely to be breech than full-term babies. In only rare cases, the breech position is associated with a birth defect, mainly a dislocated hip.

Nicole, 22, didn't find out until after she delivered her first daughter, now 2 years old, that she had a septum, or thin membrane, dividing her uterus. "But the doctor said it was very small and had nothing to do with her being breech," Nicole recalls. When her second daughter turned bottom down and stayed that way, Nicole figured it was more than a coincidence. Her babies must have been bumping up against the septum in her uterus whenever they tried to turn head-down.

Your doctor can try to feel your baby's position by placing his or her hands on your abdomen. If the baby seems to be breech, your doctor might use ultrasound to make sure. While breech babies usually don't flip late in pregnancy, head-down babies do occasionally turn breech at the last minute. More than half of the time, doctors are able to turn a breech baby and increase the chance of a vaginal delivery. In this procedure, called external cephalic (head-down) version, the doctor places his hands on mom's abdomen and pushes and rolls the baby into place. A successful version, achieved in about six out of every 10 attempts, reduces the chance of a C-section by as much as two-thirds, according to one study. Version is usually performed when the baby is full term—37 weeks or later—for two reasons: If it was done earlier, the baby might still flip back to the breech position, requiring another stab at version. And, if version were to trigger labor—one of the rare complications—the baby would not be delivered prematurely. A recent study of 232 women carrying single breech babies suggests version between 34 and 36 weeks might be even more effective and just as safe. But, the authors conclude, more research is needed before doctors routinely attempt version before 37 weeks.

Studies have found version to be safe even if you've had a prior C-section, and complications are rare. They include: your bag of waters breaking and/or labor beginning, the placenta separating from the wall of your uterus, and your baby's heart rate becoming erratic (although it usually returns to normal once the procedure is stopped).

Because there is a remote chance that your baby will need to be delivered immediately, version is performed in a hospital. Some women feel only pressure or discomfort during version, while others describe it as more painful. Research suggests that version is

TALKING POINT

If you hope to avoid a C-section, ask your doctor early in your pregnancy whether she is comfortable attempting version or delivering a breech baby vaginally.

more likely to be successful if you've had epidural anesthesia. You might also get a drug to relax your uterus and prevent contractions. Before, during, and after a version attempt, your doctor will closely monitor your baby's heart rate. If there are any problems with you or with the baby, your doctor will immediately halt the procedure. Version itself takes only 5 minutes, tops, but you might spend about 3 hours in the hospital while the epidural wears off and your doctor monitors your baby's heart rate and checks your uterus.

Ericka was planning to deliver her third baby at home, just as she had delivered her first two. But when she was about 37 weeks along, her midwives discovered that the baby was breech, and there was no way that they would try a home delivery. Fortunately for Ericka, who was determined to give birth at home, the midwives referred her to a doctor skilled at version. Even though she declined an epidural, Ericka felt only pressure, not pain. "I think I got lucky," says Ericka, now 37. It seemed like the doctor turned her baby in less than 30 seconds, and Ericka safely delivered at home 8 months ago.

Since everything she read about labor and delivery emphasized the importance of avoiding a C-section, Lisa, now 34, says she felt compelled to try version when her son turned breech 2 or 3 weeks before his due date. It didn't work, and she regrets that she even bothered. "I didn't realize until I got to the hospital that I had to be hooked up to all these monitors," she says. She delivered her son, now 3½, by a planned cesarean the following week.

Even though version carries a low risk of complications, Melanie's doctor was reluctant to try it on her. Melanie, 28, lives in Florida—land of soaring medical malpractice insurance premiums. Although complications from version are rare, her doctor had visions of a lawsuit should a problem arise. But Melanie and her husband had their hearts set on an unmedicated vaginal delivery. They went online in search of answers and learned that babies in the womb are drawn to light and to voices. So Melanie's 32-year-old husband, William, would shine a light between her legs and talk to, well, her crotch. Melanie swam just about everyday in her aunt's heated pool (even South Florida gets a tad cooler in March) in the hope that the buoyancy would prompt her daughter to flip. But at every doctor's visit, sonograms showed the baby had not budged.

Finally, her doctor agreed to try version, which was scheduled for the following Tuesday. The baby had other ideas, though. After leaking a little fluid throughout the Thursday before her version appointment, Melanie had what she describes as a "gush"—not a "TV movie gush," but a gush nonetheless, at around 11:00 P.M. Instead of calling her doctor, she decided to try to get some sleep.

Because she had not felt a torrent of fluid rush out of her body, she wasn't absolutely certain that her bag of waters had broken. After all, this was her first pregnancy, so she wasn't exactly an expert, and she "didn't want to be one of those people who goes to the hospital with every little ache and pain." Perhaps her hesitancy was wishful thinking, because her doctor had told her version was out of the question once her water broke.

By 2:00 A.M., Melanie's contractions were painful enough that she couldn't sleep. At 7:00 A.M. Friday, she finally called her doctor, who told her to go to the hospital immediately. Melanie and her husband arrived at the hospital around 8:00 A.M. A quick exam by the doctor confirmed that the baby's amniotic sac had ruptured and that her daughter was still breech. The baby was delivered by C-section at 11:21 A.M.

Despite years of seeking alternatives, researchers have

Words from the Wise

When your bag of waters breaks, don't expect Niagara Falls. Trickles are more likely than torrents.

found there's really nothing except version that can turn breech babies. Lying with your knees to your chest doesn't work. Lying on your back, a wedge-shaped cushion elevating your pelvis, doesn't work. And, probably, not even burning smelly herbs between your toes—a traditional Chinese medical practice called moxibustion—works. Only one small study, albeit a study published in the respected *Journal of the American Medical Association*, found moxibustion to be effective in turning babies. That study is frequently cited by moxibustion proponents, but no one has ever replicated its findings.

Research led by University of Toronto scientists prompted the American College of Obstetricians and Gynecologists in December 2001 to recommend cesarean delivery of breech babies who couldn't be turned by version, although that had long been standard practice. The international study included more than 2,000 women whose babies were in the breech position. Half of the women were assigned to deliver by planned C-sections, half by planned vaginal births. However, many women who were supposed to deliver vaginally ended up having a C-section because of problems that arose during labor or delivery.

"If you plan for a vaginal delivery, depending on your situation, you will run a 10 percent to 40 percent chance of having an emergency C-section," says Mary Hannah, M.D., the OB/GYN who led the breech birth study. Hannah found that to be the case when she pooled the results of her study with two other studies in which women carrying breech babies were randomly assigned to deliver vaginally or by cesarean. Of the women assigned to deliver vaginally, 45 percent needed a C-section.

Even if your doctor is willing to deliver your breech baby vaginally, you might not want to take the chance of going through a long labor and ending up with a cesarean. Although a C-section had been the furthest thing from her mind during the first 8 months of her pregnancy, Tabitha, 35, decided to schedule one when her baby wouldn't budge from the breech position after an attempted version. "I can do it this way: planned, knowing what to expect, or I can go into labor and may end up having a C-section anyway," she reasoned. "We knew the doctor who was going to deliver."

According to Hannah's study, that was probably the

> **Words from the Wise**
>
> *If your breech baby's not excessively large and your pelvis isn't exceptionally small, and if your placenta is in the right place (that is, out of the way) and you've plenty of amniotic fluid, then you might be a good candidate for a vaginal delivery in the hands of a skilled doctor.*

best approach—at least as far as breech babies are concerned. Hannah and her collaborators found that the type of delivery made no difference in the already extremely low risk of serious complications in moms. But the babies delivered by planned C-sections before labor began fared much better than those delivered vaginally. Some doctors have challenged Hannah's findings, however. For example, OB/GYN Russell Laros, M.D., of the University of California, San Francisco, says some baby deaths blamed on vaginal delivery were actually unrelated to how they were born. "I think this is an emotional, still not proven issue," Laros says of the practice to deliver all breech babies by cesarean. He continues to offer vaginal delivery of breech babies to patients in whom version was unsuccessful, as long the baby weighs less than 9 pounds and mom's pelvis appears to be large enough to accommodate such a birth. A recent study of breech births by University College Dublin researchers identified a few other criteria that improve the chances of a vaginal delivery. They include plenty of amniotic fluid, a normally formed baby, and a placenta that isn't blocking the way.

You already know from his comments above that Laros is one of a small minority of doctors still willing to deliver breech babies vaginally. Imagine how difficult it must be to find a doctor willing to do it for a woman who previously had a C-section, given the recent drop in vaginal births after cesareans, or VBACs. Nicole, who had a C-section because her first daughter was breech, assumed she'd have to go that route again when, against the odds, her second daughter turned breech 36 weeks into her pregnancy. But she found a doctor who let her try a VBAC, and after just a half-hour of pushing, her 7-pound, 4-ounce daughter was born.

If you end up scheduling a C-section because your baby is breech, the University of Toronto researchers' findings should provide some reassurance. After analyzing the immediate impact of delivery method on breech babies, the Toronto doctors checked with the mothers in their study 3 months after giving birth. They found no differences between the vaginal and cesarean delivery groups as far as breastfeeding, infant health, ease of caring for the baby, getting used to being a new mother, relationship—sexual and otherwise—with husband or partner, depression, and views about their childbirth experience. The women in the C-section group did appear to have a lower risk of urinary incontinence, but Hannah—the lead author of the study—downplays that result somewhat. She notes that she and her collaborators hadn't given the women any tips about how to reduce their risk of incontinence after delivery, such as performing Kegel exercises. And the researchers hadn't collected any information about whether the women were incontinent before delivery.

"I'm not as sure that this is a true and important finding as I would be if we had done all that. I think we need more research before we get to the point where we're recommending that women have cesareans to avoid problems with incontinence," Hannah says. "Having said that, it does provide one more bit of evidence that an elective, or planned, cesarean is not harmful in the short-term, and could be beneficial."

SUNNY SIDE UP:
THE OCCIPUT POSTERIOR POSITION

Occiput is a fancy word for the crown of the head. Normally, babies are not only head-down but also facing mom's back, a position called occiput anterior. It's ideal for birth because the baby is lined up to fit through your pelvis as smoothly as possible. Like a diver performing a cannonball, the baby's chin is tucked into his chest, which means the smallest part of his head, the crown, will press on your cervix first. After the crown stretches your cervix, it's easier for the brow—the largest part of the head—to squeeze through.

Sometimes, though, babies end up sunny-side up, facing mom's stomach. This is called the occiput posterior position. To make it through the birth canal, the baby has to turn all the way around to face mom's back. That turn happens nine out of 10 times, but it can make for a long and painful labor, which is often preceded by days or weeks of lower back pain and uncomfortable false labor.

But in one out of 10 cases, the baby never turns around to face mom's back and remains, as some put it, a stargazer. The baby is basically stuck pretty high in mom's pelvis, greatly increasing the chance of a C-section and other complications during labor and delivery. Obstetricians at Harvard's Brigham and Women's Hospital in Boston recently reported on a study of 6,434 patients who delivered full-term single babies at their hospital in 1998. The researchers excluded any pregnancy in which the mother or fetus had a condition that could influence how delivery was managed, such as diabetes in the mother or a fetus that was small for being full-term.

The doctors compared women who delivered babies in the occiput posterior position with those who delivered in the occiput anterior position. Overall, about one in 20 babies stayed face-up. The baby was more likely to remain in the occiput posterior position if she was the mother's first child. Only about a quarter of first-time moms whose babies remained sunny-side up were able to deliver vaginally. Mothers who'd previously given birth fared better. A little more than half of them were able to deliver vaginally. Among the women who delivered vaginally, mothers of babies facing up were more likely to need the assist of forceps or vacuum extraction.

In a related study, University College Dublin researchers found an even lower proportion of babies remained face-up than the Harvard scientists did. Even so, the Irish researchers concluded that babies who stayed in the occiput posterior position accounted for a sizeable 12 percent of all cesareans performed because labor failed to progress.

If your baby is face-up late in your pregnancy, a midwife might recommend that you try some of the same turning techniques as moms with breech babies, such as lying on a slant board, swimming or doing handstands in a pool, or getting on your hands and knees and slowly rocking your pelvis back and forth. Unfortunately, this advice is based mainly on personal belief or custom, not scientific evidence. In the largest study of pelvic rocking to date, Australian researchers enrolled about 2,500 women who were 37 weeks pregnant. The scientists randomly assigned half of the women to do pelvic rocking exercises for 10 minutes twice daily until they went into labor. For comparison, the other women were asked simply to walk daily. About 8 percent of the rocking mothers' babies turned sunny-side up and stayed there. And about 8 percent of the walking mothers' babies turned sunny-side up and stayed there. Pelvic rocking—not exactly the easiest exercise to perform in your last month of pregnancy—might help ease the pain of back labor, but it's not going to turn your baby around.

All is not lost, though. When your baby's head can be seen through your vaginal opening, your doctor may try to turn it with his hands or with forceps or vacuum extraction. (See chapter 5, page 126 for more about why, if you hope to deliver vaginally, it's important to find a doctor skilled in using these tools.)

SQUEEZE PLAY: BABY'S BIG, YOUR PELVIS ISN'T

The idea that pregnant women shouldn't overeat dates back to the 19th century. At the time, death rates from labor and delivery were still exceedingly high, a situation doctors blamed at least partly on babies that were too large to push out. Up until World War II, most published studies of weight gain during pregnancy reported low

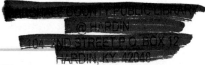

TALKING POINT

If you want to minimize your chance of having a C-section, make sure your doctor knows how to turn babies who persist in facing the wrong way. (Remember, though, a considerable number of women with babies who can't be turned are able to deliver vaginally.)

average gains, some less than 20 pounds. As recently as 1961, at least one obstetrics textbook recommended that women gain no more than 20 pounds if they wanted the best possible pregnancy outcome. But by 1976, obstetrics textbooks began recommending that pregnant women be allowed to eat and expand as much as they wanted, as insurance that their babies would be well-nourished. And most pregnant women have been all too happy to comply.

As more and more moms look at pregnancy as a license to, let's say, eat a bit too much, more and more babies are born big enough to shop for in the toddlers' department. (Okay, that might be a slight exaggeration but you get the point.) It appears that the more things change, the more they stay the same. Like their 19th-century predecessors, doctors and midwives these days are concerned about the effect of excessive weight gain during pregnancy. Generally, the more moms gain, the bigger their babies. Hefty infants can take longer to push out than smaller ones and, on rare occasions, actually get their shoulders stuck as they're trying to exit—a dangerous situation called shoulder dystocia. Shoulder dystocia can damage the nerves that control the muscles in the baby's shoulder, arm, or hand, a condition called a brachial plexus injury or Erb's Palsy. In the majority of cases, the injury heals within a few months; but, if the nerves are torn, brachial plexus injuries are permanent.

To prevent such injuries, doctors are more likely to perform C-sections if they think the baby is extra-large, but they may not really have to. According to one recent estimate, doctors would have to perform more than 3,600 C-sections in non-diabetic women suspected of carrying extra-large babies (defined below) just to prevent a single permanent birth injury in a newborn (the risk of such injuries is greater in large babies born to diabetic women. More on that later, too).

If your doctor predicts macrosomia. Large newborns are described as "macrosomic" or "large for gestational age," neither of which can be confirmed until the baby is actually delivered and weighed. Some doctors define macrosomia—literally "big body"— as a birth weight of at least 8 pounds, 12 ounces, which describes about 10 percent of U.S. newborns these days. Others, including the American College of Obstetricians and Gynecologists, consider macrosomia to be a birth weight of 9 pounds, 15 ounces or more, a size only about 1½ percent of U.S. newborns reach. Although the risks to mothers and babies begin to increase above 8 pounds, 12 ounces, they rise sharply at 9 pounds, 15 ounces and up.

"Large for gestational age" is used to describe any newborn whose birth weight is in the top 10 percent of infants of the same sex and ethnicity. Boys typically weigh more than girls at birth, and Hispanic babies are more likely to be large than white, black, or Asian babies. If you've previously delivered a baby weighing more than 8 pounds, 12 ounces, you're five to 10 times more likely to deliver a baby weighing more than 9 pounds, 15 ounces than a woman who's never delivered a large baby. If you weigh more than 300 pounds, your chance of delivering a baby who weighs 10 pounds or more is eight times greater than that of a normal-weight woman.

For another clue about your chances of delivering a large baby, ask your mother. One study found that compared to women who started out lighter in life, those who weighed more than 8 pounds at

TALKING POINT

Ask your mother how much you weighed when you were born. If you were particularly large or small, you may be more likely to deliver your own baby by C-section.

birth are twice as likely to deliver a baby weighing more than 8 pounds, 13 ounces. Your birth weight may also be related to your chances of having a cesarean, another study found. Women whose birth weight was less than 5½ pounds or greater than 8 pounds, 12 ounces were slightly more likely to have C-sections than women in the middle weight range. Perhaps the women who were smaller at birth tended to remain on the petite side as adults, while those who were heavier at birth were likely to have large babies.

As for the here and now, London researchers analyzed data from 350,000 deliveries to identify who was more likely to have a macrosomic baby, and what were the resulting risks. They found that macrosomia was more common when mom had a body mass index greater than 30 (the equivalent of a 5-foot-4-inch woman weighing at least 175 pounds), had already celebrated her 40th birthday, or had diabetes. And macrosomic babies were about twice as likely to be delivered by C-section than smaller infants.

Diagnosing a baby with macrosomia before birth is extremely imprecise. It's nearly impossible for doctors or ultrasound studies to predict whether your baby is too large to deliver vaginally—you can probably do a better job yourself! One study found that women who'd gone past their due date came just as close as their doctors did to predicting their large babies' weight. Another study found that doctors' predictions were wrong half of the time, and for good reason. As delivery approaches, your baby will descend into your pelvis, making it tricky to accurately measure his head. Plus, if your bag of waters breaks, or the level of amniotic fluid decreases, measurements may be less reliable. Macrosomic babies' sizes are especially hard to estimate. They may be so big that ultrasound can't capture the entire cross section of their abdomen or head.

Joan had gained a reasonable 25 pounds or so during her pregnancy, and her doctor figured that her daughter, now 5, would weigh about 7 pounds. But Joan ended up pushing for 4 hours before her doctor finally used forceps to extract the baby. "They said, 'Why is she having so much trouble pushing out a 7-pound baby? Then she came out. Everybody gasped when they learned her weight: 9 pounds, 10 ounces. They just really misjudged it."

If your doctor predicts macrosomia, you're more likely to deliver by cesarean. Whether it's necessary is another question, suggests a University of Louisville study of babies who weighed at least 9 pounds, 4 ounces at birth. If their macrosomia was suspected before birth, they had a 50 percent chance of being delivered by C-section. But if their macrosomia was unexpected, they had only a 30 percent chance of a cesarean birth. Why the difference? When macrosomia was predicted, doctors were more likely to induce labor.

Doctors acquired that habit because they believed they shouldn't let large babies get a whit bigger in their mothers' wombs. The problem is, inducing labor when mom's cervix isn't ready for delivery greatly increases the chance of a C-section (more on that in chapter 5, page 126). And even though they're more likely to be delivered by cesarean, babies whose macrosomia was predicted are no less likely to get stuck or even injured than big babies who fooled their moms' doctors, research suggests. That's why the American College of Obstetricians and Gynecologists (ACOG) recommends

---

TALKING POINT

Even if your doctor thinks your baby is big, but you're not diabetic (more on that later), you should be allowed to try to deliver vaginally—as long as your labor progresses at a reasonable pace, and the baby's heart rate is reassuring, according to ACOG.

---

against labor induction or preplanned C-sections simply because a baby is thought to be macrosomic before birth. **If your doctor predicts cephalopelvic disproportion.** Another term you might have heard in reference to large babies is cephalopelvic disproportion, which simply means that the baby's head is thought to be too big to fit through the mother's pelvis. A whopping 96.5 percent of women diagnosed with cephalopelvic disproportion end up having C-sections. One study found that women whose mothers delivered them by cesarean because of cephalopelvic disproportion or dysfunctional labor were more likely to deliver their own babies by cesarean.

But unless your pelvis is abnormally small, say, because of injuries from a car wreck or it's just your particular anatomy, you are not necessarily destined to have a C-section if your baby is large. You have to remember that during labor, your pelvis expands and your baby's skull—made up of five plates connected by soft tissue— is pliable. That's why so many temporarily look like cone heads, a souvenir of their trip through the birth canal. If your doctor suspects that your baby and your pelvis are a mismatch size-wise, she might suggest measuring your pelvis, usually using x-ray. However, a review of four studies totaling more than 1,000 women found that this

TALKING POINT

If your doctor wants to x-ray your pelvis to see if it's big enough to accommodate your baby, press her for an explanation. While it's unlikely that the findings will affect your baby either way, they could increase your chances of having a C-section.

technique, called x-ray pelvimetry, did not appear to have a significant impact on how babies fared. But the women who underwent pelvimetry were twice as likely to be delivered by cesarean than women whose pelvis wasn't x-rayed.

Nanci is 4-foot-10-inches . . . barely. "For my first daughter's birth, I went through 7 hours of labor that was induced, but I made very little progress," she says. After delivering her first daughter by unplanned cesarean, she figured it wasn't even worth trying to deliver her second baby vaginally, so she scheduled a C-section. To this day, she doesn't believe that there's any way a woman as petite as she is could vaginally deliver babies as big as hers: Her firstborn, now 16, weighed 8 pounds; her second, now 13, nearly that. "Both had large heads," remembers Nanci, 46. "In fact, when my second daughter was born, I said, 'Look at the head on that baby,' and the obstetrician said, 'Well, I didn't want to say anything, but it is large.' "

If you have diabetes and your doctor predicts macrosomia. The situation gets a little more complicated if you have diabetes, one of the

Looking Back

Let's clear up one common misconception right now: Julius Caesar's mother most likely did not deliver him via cesarean section. It made a good story, though, one that persisted through the centuries. In Caesar's time and for centuries afterward, C-sections were mainly used as last-ditch efforts to save the baby of a mom who had died or wasn't going to make it through childbirth. Doctors simply didn't know enough about human anatomy and physiology to expect both mother and baby to survive the operation. According to Caesar's writings, his mom, Aurelia, was still alive when he invaded Britain, so there's only a very remote possibility that she had delivered him by C-section.

main risk factors for macrosomia. If you developed diabetes after you became pregnant, a condition called gestational diabetes, you're three to four times more likely to have a C-section than the general population. If your diabetes predates your pregnancy, your chance of having a cesarean delivery is even higher.

Research suggests that macrosomic babies of diabetic mothers tend to be shaped differently—read: harder to push out—than macrosomic babies of non-diabetic mothers. The diabetic mothers' babies tend to have greater total body fat, be bigger around the arms and shoulders, and have larger heads in relationship to their abdomens. So even among macrosomic babies who weigh the same, those born to diabetic mothers have a greater chance of shoulder dystocia, and with it, a greater risk of permanent injury. If you are diabetic and your baby appears to be large, your doctor should discuss the possibility of a preplanned cesarean delivery. In addition to your baby's estimated weight, your doctor should consider two other major factors when deciding whether to recommend a C-section: your obstetrical history (such as whether you've ever delivered vaginally) and what a pelvic exam says about your readiness for a vaginal delivery.

But some studies suggest that doctors are more likely to want to perform cesareans simply because a patient has diabetes. For example, a review of more than 42,000 births in South Carolina found higher rates of C-sections among diabetic women who had no other indications for one. In other words, their babies were of normal size and they had no medical conditions other than diabetes that might predispose them to a cesarean.

HARD LABOR: TIME MIGHT BE EVERYTHING

"Failure to progress" in labor is a common reason for unplanned C-sections. Sometimes, though, it may simply be failure to wait.

TALKING POINT

It's difficult to estimate a baby's size before birth. If you have diabetes and your doctor recommends a C-section because your baby is large, press for an explanation.

Studies suggest that some doctors and patients can be too quick to abandon plans for a vaginal delivery. Those judgment calls help explain why C-section rates vary so much from hospital to hospital and doctor to doctor. For example, if you deliver at South Miami Hospital in Florida, you're more than five times more likely to end up having a C-section than if you're admitted to Zuni–Ramah Hospital in northwestern New Mexico.

In 1996, just over 7 percent of the babies born at Zuni–Ramah were delivered by cesarean. That same year, the U.S. C-section rate was nearly 21 percent. The hospital's amazingly low C-section rate occurred in a population of Zuni and Navajo women who had high rates of diabetes and preeclampsia, both risk factors for C-sections. What was going on here? Lawrence Leeman, one of the family practice doctors who delivers babies at Zuni–Ramah, and his wife, Rebecca Leeman, a certified nurse midwife, uncovered two main reasons for the hospital's low rate of cesareans. Because so few women delivered their first babies by cesarean, fewer were having repeat C-sections. Makes sense. The other main reason for Zuni–Ramah's low C-section rate: First-time mothers were only about a fifth as likely as their counterparts nationwide to undergo a cesarean for dystocia, which simply means slow or difficult labor. Dystocia is a catchall for a variety of problems. Mom's pelvis might be too small or her uterine contractions too few or too weak to cause her cervix to dilate properly. The baby might be too big or in the wrong position like Annie's son, who turned breech at the last minute. There could be a combination of these factors. Or the only problem might simply be a lack of patience on the part of the doctor and, sometimes, the mother herself.

Dystocia is thought to account for 30 percent of all C-sections in the United States, including as many as half of those performed on first-time mothers. If you consider that many women who deliver their first baby by cesarean end up scheduling repeat C-sections, the diagnosis of dystocia might be at least indirectly related to 50 to 60 percent of all cesareans.

Maybe the problem lies not with the women diagnosed with dystocia but with how doctors define the term. Women today are held to a half-century-old labor standard called the Friedman curve, one of the first things obstetrics students learn in their training.

Emanuel Friedman wasn't yet 30 when he plotted the eponymous scale in 1953, during his residency training in obstetrics and gynecology in New York. Friedman found that, on average, it took 2½ hours for the cervix to dilate from 4 to 10 centimeters.

"In the last 50 years, the Friedman curve pretty much dictated obstetric practice, at least in the United States," says Jun Zhang, Ph.D., an epidemiologist at the National Institute for Child Health and Human Development, part of the National Institutes of Health.

It's been 13 years since Betsy, 48, delivered her second daughter, but she'll never forget how her obstetrician whipped out a graph of the Friedman scale while she was in labor to demonstrate that it was time to give up her goal of a VBAC and agree to her second C-section.

Several reports suggest that many cesareans performed for dystocia might be unnecessary. When labor appears to be stalled, doctors—as well as patients—often give up too quickly and move on to a C-section. For example, a study of deliveries at 30 Los Angeles and Iowa hospitals found that about a quarter of women who had cesareans for lack of progress were only in the very first phase of labor, called the latent phase, when the procedure was performed. Some hadn't even begun to dilate. That doesn't square with the American College of Obstetricians and Gynecologists' definition of dystocia: no dilation of the cervix and no descent of the baby for at least 2 hours during *active* labor.

The first stage of active labor generally begins when your cervix is dilated to about 4 centimeters and ends when it is fully dilated to 10 centimeters. The second stage of active labor is when you begin to push. In the Los Angeles/Iowa study, more than a third of the women who had C-sections after they were fully dilated hadn't been pushing an exceptionally long time, as far as ACOG guidelines are concerned. (According to those guidelines, a "prolonged second stage of labor" is one that lasts more than 3 hours in any woman who's had an epidural or 1 or 2 hours—depending on whether she's a first-time mom—in a woman who didn't get an epidural.) Maybe, the researchers suggest, doctors have become so comfortable performing C-sections that they've relaxed their definition of lack of progress in labor.

Zuni-Ramah, on the other hand, isn't even equipped to do cesarean deliveries. If two doctors agree that a C-section is needed, the patient must be transported to a bigger hospital 35 miles away. The Leemans speculate that the logistics of obtaining a C-section motivate doctors and patients to wait out slow labor. Such an approach apparently hasn't caused an excess number of problems in either babies or mothers at Zuni-Ramah.

Research by Zhang and others suggests that the Friedman scale has not kept up with the times. Far more women are getting epidurals, and they're putting on more pounds than ever during pregnancy—both factors that can slow labor. For example, researchers from the University of Texas Southwestern Medical Center at Dallas found that the active stage of labor averaged an hour longer in patients assigned to get an epidural, compared to those assigned to get an intravenous narcotic painkiller. The Dallas study was a randomized controlled trial, considered the gold standard of patient research. In this trial, 459 first-time mothers were randomly assigned to receive either an epidural or an intravenous narcotic painkiller. There was no difference in the groups' C-section rates, which were so low that some doctors questioned whether that particular finding could be applied to laboring women in general.

You don't need a randomized trial to know that moms, and, therefore, their babies, have grown increasingly heavier over the last half century. "Mother's weight has a direct effect on baby size," Zhang says. "The babies are getting bigger. That's not just in the U.S., but also in other countries. The bigger baby not only means slower labor, but also a higher C-section rate. The question is, how much is that due to the big baby, or how much is due to the expectation that labor is supposed to go fast, but it didn't? Maybe physicians are too quick to make a diagnosis of dystocia." Catherine Spong, M.D., head of perinatology research at the National Insti-

TALKING POINT

If you hope to deliver vaginally, let your doctor know that you're willing to ride out a long labor as long as you and your baby are doing fine. Then she won't rush in to perform a C-section.

tute of Child Health and Human Development, says she learned a valuable lesson while training to be an OB/GYN: "If you were patient enough, most babies could come out vaginally."

To determine when performing a C-section is more beneficial than allowing a woman to continue to labor, Zhang hopes to collect information about cervical dilation and labor progression on 200,000 deliveries nationwide. He's already done some research that backs up his theory that doctors are often too hasty. Zhang and two colleagues examined detailed labor data for more than 1,300 first-time mothers. The women were not induced, and they delivered full-term, head-down babies vaginally. Sure enough, it took the women an average of 5½ hours to progress from 4 to 10 centimeters—more than twice as long as what Friedman observed in the early 1950s. Before the women in Zhang's study reached 7 centimeters, it wasn't uncommon for dilation to stall for more than 2 hours, which fits the American College of Obstetricians and Gynecologists' criteria for too-slow labor. In other words, these women were prime C-section candidates, who, for whatever reason, were allowed to continue to labor and deliver vaginally without any problem.

"The earlier stage of labor is naturally very slow," says Zhang. So if you're doing fine, and your baby's doing fine, there's no reason to rush to a C-section just because you're hung up at 4 or 5 centimeters. It's a different story if you stall later, though. "If you're stuck for 2 hours at 9 centimeters, you should probably have a C-section," Zhang says. "That is truly stuck."

Words from the Wise

When you're dilated just a few centimeters, labor can be slow-going. If you become frustrated with what you perceive as a lack of progress, you might be setting yourself up for a C-section.

TWICE AS NICE: DELIVERING TWINS

Just because you're carrying two babies doesn't necessarily mean you'll have a C-section, although half of all twins are delivered that way. If both babies are head-down, you should expect to be able to deliver vaginally, according to the American College of Obstetricians and Gynecologists. Most researchers agree that if both twins are head-down, vaginal delivery is appropriate after 33 weeks gestation or if the babies each weigh at least 3 pounds, 5 ounces. Although there's not exactly a plethora of research to suggest that smaller, more premature twins should be delivered via C-section, that has become a common practice.

In 60 percent of all twin pregnancies, at least one of the babies is breech. If the first twin to be delivered is breech, ACOG recommends that you have a cesarean delivery, but it acknowledges that scientific opinion on the matter is split.

To determine whether a planned C-section or a vaginal delivery was better for twins, University of Toronto researchers recently pooled the results of four studies, totaling more than 1,900 infants, then compared the two different modes of birth. The only possible benefit they found to delivering twins by cesarean was a decreased chance of a low Apgar score 5 minutes after birth, particu-

TALKING POINT

Don't assume you have to deliver twins by C-section. If you want to try to deliver them vaginally, make sure that your doctor is comfortable with the idea early in your pregnancy.

larly if the first twin delivered was breech. The Apgar test rates your baby's skin color, breathing, muscle tone, reflexes and pulse at 1 minute and 5 minutes after birth. It was designed to assess whether a newborn needs immediate attention, such as extra help with breathing. A low score (below 7 on a 10-point scale) seldom indicates any long-term problems. The study's bottom line: It's not worth undergoing a C-section just to raise your baby's 5-minute Apgar score.

Some doctors who specialize in treating incontinence believe that delivering twins by planned C-section carries an additional benefit, that of lowering the chance of urine leakage and other pelvic floor problems down the road. However, the research is far from conclusive.

What if your second twin isn't head down? Second babies in twin pregnancies are more likely to experience complications during birth, especially if they're not in that optimal head-down position. But there have been practically no randomized trials to determine whether a scheduled C-section is any safer than a vaginal delivery for second twins. One small study of 60 women concluded that delivering a breech second twin by cesarean had no obvious benefit for the baby and increased mom's risk of infections. Besides, if your second twin is breech, she might just turn head down after her sibling is delivered. If she doesn't, your doctor might try external or internal version, in which he'll put one hand through your dilated cervix and the other on your abdomen to try to turn the baby. If the baby still doesn't flip and must be delivered even more quickly than a C-section would allow, your doctor may reach into the birth canal to position her better, a technique called breech extraction. You have to remember that breech second twins have a couple of advantages over single breech babies when it comes to vaginal delivery: Twins tend to be smaller than single babies, so it's a little easier for

Words from the Wise

Even if your second twin is breech, you likely can still deliver vaginally. For a number of reasons, breech second twins are easier to deliver vaginally than single breech babies.

them to exit. And your breech second twin will have a head start—no pun intended—on a vaginal delivery, thanks to the (barely) older sibling who paved the way by widening your cervix with his head.

Even if your babies are head-down, you—like women carrying a single head-down baby—could end up delivering both or even just one by cesarean. And if you conceived them by in vitro fertilization, your chances of have a C-section might be even higher, according to recent research by doctors at the American University of Beirut in Lebanon. In their study, 77 percent of in vitro twins were delivered by cesarean, compared to 58 percent of twins conceived without the help of in vitro fertilization. Researchers at the University of Mississippi Medical Center reviewed all 106 sets of head-down twins born at their hospital over a 4-year period. In 21 sets, both babies were delivered by C-section. In 68 sets, both babies were delivered vaginally.

And in the remaining 17 cases, the mothers had the very special experience of delivering the first twin vaginally and the second by cesarean. Now that wasn't just because the second twin was dawdling in utero or—as one mother of twins born vaginally nearly half a day apart put it—had swum upstream. For the most part, doctors are no longer following the old "30-minute interval rule" in twin deliveries. In the past, doctors would routinely deliver a second twin by C-section if more than a half hour passed after the first twin was born vaginally. These days, as long as fetal monitoring shows the second twin is okay, doctors will let women

TALKING POINT

If delivering both babies vaginally is important to you, tell your doctor you're willing to wait for a slow-poke twin to make his way out, as long as you and the baby are doing fine.

continue to labor for hours past the birth their of first twin. Most of the cesareans in the Mississippi study were performed because of some apparent emergency, such as fetal distress or placenta abruptio. And in four cases, the second twin flipped out of position after the first baby's birth.

PLACENTA PROBLEMS: WHEN IT DOESN'T GROW RIGHT

To many women, one of the most mysterious parts of pregnancy is the development of what is essentially a "disposable" organ, the placenta. That special tissue provides your baby with oxygen, water, and nutrients from your blood and secretes the hormones you need for a successful pregnancy. But in most cases, it's delivered after your baby and discarded while you're blissfully cuddling with your newborn.

There's not much that you can do to affect the normal growth of the placenta and you probably don't give yours a second thought. But it's so important that it even merits its own eponymous medical journal, *Placenta*. (Just *Placenta*. Ranks right up there with *Chest* and *Gut*.) Still, as important as the placenta is, it's also the center of a C-section catch 22: Placenta abnormalities increase your risk of having a C-section, while having a C-section increases your risk of placenta abnormalities.

Even with access to the top obstetrical care the British Empire has to offer, Sophie, Countess of Wessex, still experienced a placenta problem that necessitated an emergency C-section 5 weeks before her due date in late 2003. That development took both her family, including mother-in-law Queen Elizabeth, and her doctors by surprise. Sophie's husband, Edward, the queen's youngest child, wasn't even in the country when she delivered their firstborn, a daughter who is eighth in line for the throne.

Reportedly, Sophie experienced a complication called placenta abruptio, in which the placenta peels away from the uterus and cuts off the flow of oxygen to the baby. Only a small percentage of cases have a definable cause. They include an auto accident or a fall, a sudden collapse of the uterus as amniotic fluid rushes out, delivery of a first twin, or an abnormally short umbilical cord. Risk factors for placenta abruptio include advanced maternal age—at 38, sad to say, Sophie qualified—placenta abruptio in a previous pregnancy and high blood pressure. If the mother is bleeding, as Sophie was, or monitoring shows signs of fetal distress, a C-section is often the preferred mode of delivery. (By the way, Sophie and daughter Louise Alice Elizabeth Mary Mountbatten-Windsor—whew!—were doing fine at last report.)

Sometimes the placenta grows in the wrong place. In a condition called placenta previa, which occurs in about one out of every 200 births, the placenta makes itself at home in the lower part of the uterus, blocking baby's exit. Your risk of placenta previa is even higher if you're 35 or older, are carrying more than one baby, or have delivered several children already. If you've had six or more previous deliveries, your risk could be as high as one in 20. You're

TALKING POINT

Call your doctor or midwife immediately if you experience vaginal bleeding (we're not talking about just light spotting here) in your second or third trimester. It could be a sign of a problem with your placenta. If you can't reach your caregiver, go to the nearest emergency room.

also at increased risk if you've had fibroids removed through an incision in your uterus or a previous C-section scar is very low in the uterus. Spotting in the first trimester, and bleeding in the second or third or during labor, are the main symptoms—although your doctor can spot a low-lying placenta on ultrasound during the second trimester. Placenta previa is a cesarean success story, as the operation has greatly reduced deaths of mothers and babies from this condition. Of the women diagnosed with placenta previa in 2001, 81 percent delivered via C-section.

THROUGH THE ROOF:
HIGH BLOOD PRESSURE COULD HIKE
YOUR CHANCES OF A C-SECTION

The only cure for pregnancy-induced high blood pressure, or preeclampsia, is delivery of the baby. Also called toxemia, preeclampsia affects about one out of 20 pregnant women, usually those having their first baby. It generally develops after the 20th week of pregnancy, and in addition to high blood pressure, its symptoms include swelling of the face, hands, and feet and the presence of protein in the urine. Scientists are not sure what causes preeclampsia, although they know that it tends to run in families and occurs more frequently in women with diabetes. In its most severe form, preeclampsia can damage the mother's organs and restrict the baby's growth. Preeclampsia can also increase the risk of placenta abruptio. Doctors usually prescribe bed rest until the baby has matured enough to be delivered, either by labor induction or by cesarean. In their search for ways to prevent preeclampsia, researchers have tested aspirin, calcium supplements, and magnesium, to name a few, but they've found minimal benefit, if any. Studies suggest that you can reduce your chance of developing preeclampsia by getting down to a healthy weight before pregnancy through diet and exercise. If you have high blood pressure or diabetes before you conceive, you should consult a doctor about how best to ensure a healthy pregnancy.

If you develop preeclampsia, the type of hospital where you deliver could affect how you deliver. Using Missouri birth certificate data, researchers at Saint Louis University analyzed C-section rates for more than 13,000 women with preeclampsia who had delivered their first baby. After accounting for how far along the women were when they delivered and the weight of their newborns, the researchers found that those who gave birth at a tertiary hospital were least likely to have a cesarean. Tertiary hospitals, generally academic

Words from the Wise

Some experts think that the most important prenatal visit is one that takes place before you even get pregnant, especially if you have health problems such as high blood pressure or diabetes. At a preconception appointment, your doctor can help you lay the foundation for a healthy pregnancy.

medical centers, offer the most specialized care for pregnant women and their babies. At these hospitals, 30 percent of first-time mothers with preeclampsia had C-sections, compared to 38 percent at smaller community hospitals. (See chapter 5, page 126, for more about differences in C-section rates between the two types of hospitals.)

At 30 weeks into her pregnancy, Susan M. had just started seeing her obstetrician weekly. Her feet and ankles were very swollen, and she had a lot of protein in her urine. When medication failed to control her blood pressure, a decision was made to perform an emergency cesarean. Susan's daughter weighed just 2¾ pounds, but "She was fine. She was little; she needed some time to grow. She came out screaming." Although she did grieve briefly over the loss of her dream birth experience, "the overwhelming feeling was just of gratitude that we could come through it and everything was okay."

OUTBREAK: WHEN HERPES OR OTHER INFECTIOUS DISEASES COMPLICATE MATTERS

Living with an infectious disease can be traumatic. But you can take comfort that the chances of passing it on to your baby during a vaginal delivery are lower than ever, thanks to recent advancements in preventative drug treatments. That's a good thing, because a cesarean delivery doesn't always prevent mother-to-child transmission of infectious diseases such as herpes

If you have herpes. Nearly one out of every three American women are infected with herpes, but the vast majority—one expert puts the proportion at 90 percent—don't know it. Infected mothers can transmit herpes to their babies, for whom it's a life-threatening disease.

Your risk of infecting your baby depends on when you were infected, and whether you're having an outbreak when you go into labor. The majority of pregnant women with herpes contracted the disease long before they got pregnant. Genital herpes can remain dormant for years before symptoms appear. Even then, many women mistake the itchiness and sores for an allergy to condoms or sperm, or a yeast infection. (Men can be pretty clueless as well. They often blame genital herpes symptoms on jock itch, zipper burn, or acne.) The symptoms of a herpes outbreak clear up in 3 days, just about as long as it takes medication to cure a yeast infection.

If you've been infected for years, even unknowingly, you've developed antibodies to keep the disease in check, antibodies that you pass on to your baby. So your risk of infecting your baby is far lower than that of a newly infected mother. In fact, if you have no sores or symptoms when in labor, your chance of transmitting the disease to your baby during a vaginal delivery is about 1 in 5,000. If you do have signs of an outbreak when you're in labor, your chance of passing on the disease rises considerably, to roughly 1 in 30.

About 2 percent of the 1.6 million Americans who contract herpes each year are pregnant at the time. That's fewer than 1 percent of all women in the United States who give birth annually. Because their immune systems haven't had a chance to make antibodies against the disease, they have a 50–50 chance of infecting their babies if—and that's a big if—they're having an outbreak when they go into labor.

Considering that millions of women are infected, the number of newborn cases of herpes is remarkably small. Each year in the United States, about 1,500 to 2,000 newborns are diagnosed with the disease, and most contracted it near the time of delivery. That observation led doctors to believe that they could prevent transmission by delivering mothers with outbreaks via C-sections, which then became the "standard of care" more than 30 years ago.

The American College of
Obstetricians and Gynecologists (ACOG) made it official
in 1999 with a practice bulletin on the subject. However, 20 to 30 percent of
newborns infected by herpes

Words from the Wise

*You don't have to schedule a
C-section just because you have
herpes.*

are delivered by cesarean, raising questions about its effectiveness
in halting transmission, says Deborah Cohan, M.D., an OB/GYN
at the University of California, San Francisco. Instead of performing C-sections on women having a herpes outbreak around
the time of delivery, Cohan and others recommend that doctors
should prescribe medications to prevent outbreaks in the first place.

Despite the practice's long history, the first study to demonstrate that C-sections reduce the risk of transmission from mother
to newborn was just published in 2003. The 17-year study included
58,352 women who delivered at five hospitals in Washington state.
Of that total, only 202 were found to have the herpes virus in their
genital secretions. Of those women, 117 delivered vaginally and 85
underwent C-sections. Only one of the babies delivered by cesarean contracted herpes, compared to nine of the babies who were
delivered vaginally.

Although the study was massive, it had too few cases of
herpes-infected babies to demonstrate that C-sections were indeed
beneficial for women with infections that predated their pregnancies, says Cohan, who specializes in infectious diseases during pregnancy. Perhaps the risk of transmission in these women was so low
that the researchers needed many more patients to show that cesareans do protect babies, Cohan says. If that's the case, Cohan asks,
why subject all women with active herpes to cesareans? She and her
colleagues at the medical school have decided not to. In other parts

of the world, such as the Netherlands, doctors don't routinely perform C-sections on women having a herpes outbreak in labor, and they have not seen an upswing in cases of the disease in newborns, Cohan notes.

Although University of Washington OB/GYN Zane Brown, M.D., lead author of the 2003 study, is convinced that cesareans can save the lives of babies born to women with herpes outbreaks, his hospital hasn't had to perform one for that reason in more than a decade. That's because at their first prenatal visit, virtually all pregnant women in the Seattle area are tested to see if their blood contains herpes antibodies. If it does, they'll receive a prescription for one of two antiviral medications to take during the last month of their pregnancy. Acyclovir is generic, so it's cheaper than its cousin, valacyclovir (Valtrex). But valacyclovir needs to be taken only twice a day, a dosing schedule that's a little bit easier to follow than acyclovir's three-times-a-day dosing. Neither drug has been found to have any ill effect on fetuses, Brown says, although acyclovir has a longer track record. The Acyclovir in Pregnancy Registry, which collected data about more than 1,200 pregnant women who had taken the drug, was recently closed after researchers found no increases in drug-related fetal abnormalities. The registry did not follow the babies to see if any acyclovir-related problems showed up after birth.

Antiviral drugs must do more than reduce the chance of a having an outbreak near delivery. They need to cut the amount of herpes virus in infected women's genital secretions, whether the disease is active or not. That's because women can transmit genital herpes to their newborns even when they're not having an outbreak. In fact, in 7 out of 10 cases of newborns with herpes, mothers had no symptoms around the time of delivery, but the virus was found in their genital secretions. The good news, Brown says, is that taking an antiviral drug during the last month of pregnancy cuts the risk of having herpes virus in genital secretions from 20 percent to just 5 or 6 percent. A recent article in the ACOG journal supports Brown's observation. The authors pooled the results of five studies in which a total of 799 infected women were randomly assigned to get either acyclovir or a placebo in the latter part of their pregnancies. Individually, the studies found that the women who took acyclovir were less likely to have a herpes outbreak or have a symptomless virus in their genital secretions during labor. But four of the five studies were too small to conclude with certainty that the finding was due to the drug, not to chance. By combining the studies' results, though, the researchers showed that taking acyclovir late in pregnancy really cuts infected women's risk of not only having a herpes outbreak at delivery, but also of having herpes virus in their genital secretions at that time. And compared to women taking a placebo, those on acyclovir were 70 percent less likely to have a C-section. While 55 of the 375 women given a placebo had cesarean deliveries, only 17 of 424 on acyclovir did.

TALKING POINT

Tell your doctor early in your pregnancy if you know you have herpes. If you think you might, but you're not sure, ask to be tested. Taking an antiviral medication in your last month of pregnancy can greatly reduce the chance that you'll pass the disease on to your baby at delivery.

Spurred by the research findings, Brown has become a man with a mission. "My big schtick is to go around the country to convince every woman that she should have an antibody test for genital herpes at the first prenatal visit," he says. Among Brown's mostly white, upper middle-class pregnant patients, 55 percent test positive for herpes antibodies. Still, some OB/GYNs are skeptical about the value of universal testing for genital herpes. They point out that adding a new test to every pregnant woman's first prenatal visit, even a relatively inexpensive test like the one for genital herpes, is a huge investment for what appears to be very little gain (although Brown says he has unpublished data showing that universal testing for genital herpes is cost-effective).

Hepatitis C. As far as hepatitis C, another serious viral infection that can be transmitted during delivery, "the jury is still out," Cohan says. "But, that being said, there's some very preliminary evidence that a C-section may prevent transmission of hepatitis C from mother to baby." Cohan is not routinely offering cesareans to women with hepatitis C, but she wouldn't be surprised if further research reveals that they do reduce the chance that mothers with high amounts of the virus in their blood would infect their babies.

TALKING POINT

If you have hepatitis C, discuss your delivery options with your doctor. It's not yet clear whether a planned cesarean would reduce your baby's risk of contracting the disease.

Genital warts. If you have genital warts when you go into labor, your risk of transmitting the disease to your baby is not great enough to warrant a cesarean delivery, according to the Association

> **Words from the Wise**
>
> *Just because you have genital warts doesn't mean that you have to schedule a C-section.*

of Reproductive Health Professionals. You can transmit human papillomavirus (or HPV) strains that cause genital warts to your baby during the birth process, but this is not common. Most doctors do not believe that the risk to the baby of acquiring laryngeal papillomatosis (HPV-induced warts in the voicebox or windpipe) is great enough to justify delivery by cesarean section of women who have genital warts at the time of delivery.

HIV. If you're infected with the human immunodeficiency virus, or HIV, the delivery decision gets more complicated. Planned cesareans performed before labor begins effectively protect the baby against transmission by women with high HIV levels. However, if your immune system isn't functioning normally, you face a greater risk of infection from surgery, including C-section, than healthy women. A recent study of Italian women who had cesarean deliveries found that two-thirds of the HIV-positive mothers had a complicated recovery after the operation. They were more likely to experience both major and minor postoperative complications, such as urinary tract infection and pneumonia. On average, they remained in the hospital for a week, compared to 4 days for C-section patients who weren't HIV-positive.

Fortunately, research has shown that aggressive treatment with a combination of antiviral medications during pregnancy can greatly lower women's levels of HIV, cutting the chance of transmission

Words from the Wise

If you're infected with HIV, aggressive treatment with antiviral medications can greatly lower the levels of the virus in your body, paving the way for a safe vaginal delivery.

during a vaginal delivery to less than 2 percent. In women with low levels of HIV, there is little evidence that the benefits of a C-section outweigh the risks. Still, ACOG recommends that doctors offer C-sections to all HIV-infected women. According to the OB/GYN group, the procedure should be performed 2 weeks before the due date to minimize the chance that the mother might go into labor or have her bag of waters break beforehand.

Now that you've weighed your chances for having a C-section, let's take a look at what the operation entails.

CHAPTER 2

ON THE BIG DAY

What happens in the hospital before, during, and after a C-Section

Andrea has some advice for any mom who ends up having a C-section: Don't get all righteous and refuse the painkillers they offer to you in the hospital afterward.

Andrea had already dealt with far more medical interventions than she ever expected with the birth of her first child, a daughter who's now 2½. She'd been induced. She'd had a C-section. So no heavy-duty painkillers afterward, thank you very much. "I had this notion while in the hospital that I just shouldn't take narcotics," recalls Andrea, 39. "That was a really bad call on my part." Her incision hurt, so her resolve not to use narcotics didn't last long.

Andrea thinks a little forewarning about what it's like to have a C-section would have helped her recovery. She would have liked to know beforehand exactly how it was going to feel and how to best manage the pain.

Because she developed a fever during labor that didn't subside until 5 days later, Andrea spent a week in the hospital. Another 2 or 3 weeks passed before she could move like a normal person. "You feel happy, but you're exhausted. The saving grace was that it was right after Election Day. There was a lot of interesting stuff on CNN."

Although her delivery didn't turn out as she'd expected, Andrea is grateful that her doctor had a C-section in his back pocket when it appeared that a vaginal birth wasn't meant to be. "My daughter came out perfect," *Andrea says.*

No one is crazy about the idea of undergoing surgery. But knowing what to expect can help lessen your anxiety. Since most women who end up having C-sections weren't expecting one, it's a good idea to familiarize yourself with the procedure. This chapter will walk you through it, from the time you set foot in the hospital until the time you're wheeled out (a wheelchair exit is standard even for women who deliver vaginally), your snoozing baby snuggled in your arms.

Gigi learned everything she knows about C-sections from personal experience. She's had four of them. Now 42, she was 24 when she had her first and only unplanned cesarean. "I remember thinking that childbirth would be a breeze, and when my water broke, I showered, blew-dry my hair, applied makeup and nail polish and packed a bottle of champagne so that my husband and I could celebrate in the hospital. Little did I know that 4 hours later my nail polish would be scrubbed off, my makeup would be streaming, awash in tears, and my hair would be matted to my head . . . in short, Regan from *The Exorcist* in the early stages of possession. No more thoughts of champagne or celebration."

Not to worry, though. By the time her son was delivered, Gigi had concluded that cesarean was the only way to deliver. "I decided then and there that I wouldn't mind having more kids as long as I could opt for C-sections," she says. "The operation itself was so fast and efficient that I felt amazed that it could all be over so quickly."

At her second cesarean, Gigi was the epitome of calm. "During the operation, the doctors, my husband and I critiqued who was the best anchorwoman—Jane Pauley or Deborah Norville," she recalls. "By childbirth number four, I was pretty much running the show."

Cynthia took a novel approach to dealing with the unfamiliar sights of the operating room when she delivered twins, her only children, by cesarean. If she could have, she would have skipped delivery and gone right to holding her babies. The next best thing, Cynthia decided, was to shut her eyes until it was over. From the time she was being wheeled into surgery until the time someone in the operating room held her babies up to her face, Cynthia didn't see a thing. "I didn't want any memories of this brightly lit, sterile room with 50 people running around," she explains. Her twins are now 3 months old, and Cynthia, who's in her 40s, has no regrets about not even taking a peek. On the other hand, some women find the experience so fascinating that they watch the whole operation, thanks to a properly positioned mirror above them.

It's unlikely there were really 50 people in Cynthia's operating room, as she would have known if she'd had the chance to learn about C-sections beforehand. If, like Cynthia, you know that you're definitely going to deliver by that route, check to see if any local hospitals offer classes in cesarean preparation. A typical class focuses on coping techniques, such as slow-paced breathing to help relax before surgery. You'll also learn about comfortable positions for breastfeeding after having a C-section. And you and your husband or other support person will learn what to expect in the cold, noisy operating room.

Words from the Wise

Look into whether your hospital offers a cesarean preparation class. Doctors and nurses say women who end up having an unplanned C-section tend to cope better with the pain and recover more quickly if they've had advance preparation.

BEFORE YOU GO: WHAT TO PACK

Even if you're scheduled to be induced or have a C-section, you might not want to wait until the very last minute to pack your hospital bag. It's possible that your bag of waters could break or contractions might begin before your hospital appointment.

Some basics:

- Comfy slippers, socks, underwear, and a bathrobe. Leave nightgowns and your silk robe at home—the first few days after you give birth, whether by C-section or not, can be a little messy. (Yeah, those hospital gowns aren't exactly stylish—but hey, you won't have to worry about laundering them.)
- Receiving blanket and going-home outfit for the baby
- Toiletries and cosmetics
- Magazines or other reading material for when the baby is sleeping
- Change for vending machines
- Film or digital camera. (The fun thing about digital photos is that your husband or other friend or relative will be able to e-mail them across the country before you even leave the hospital.)
- Video camera, if you have one. (Remember, some hospitals and/or doctors won't let you tape the actual birth because of liability concerns.)
- Cell phone
- Non-perishable snacks for you and your partner. If you become ravenous after delivering vaginally at 2:00 A.M., you may be disappointed to find that the hospital kitchen and cafeteria are closed until breakfast. (For more on why you may not be allowed to eat right away, see "Fine dining: No reason to starve after a C-section," on page 66.)

- Personal stereo with headphones or a portable stereo and a selection of your favorite music to deliver by
- Earplugs to block out hospital chatter and clatter so you can sleep at night
- Nursing bras, if you're going to breastfeed
- List of names and phone numbers of people you'll want to call after the baby's birth

For convenience, you could wear the same clothes to and from the hospital. Don't expect to zip up your skinny jeans as soon as you deliver. The best you'll probably be able to do is to fit into clothes you wore toward the end of your second trimester. It takes about 6 weeks for your uterus to shrink back to its pre-pregnancy size. And, as you've probably guessed by now, you won't immediately lose every single one of those pregnancy pounds when you give birth—unless you deliver a 20-pound baby!

THE ABCs OF C-SECTIONS: FROM START TO FINISH

If you arrive at the hospital during regular business hours, whether in labor or to undergo a planned C-section, you'll probably go in through the main entrance. Depending on your hospital, you'll then either go to admitting or to the maternity unit (you should have pre-registered—many hospitals even provide downloadable forms on their Web sites). If you arrive at the hospital in the middle of the night, you might enter through the emergency department instead of the main entrance. You can learn all about where to go and who to see (not to mention where to park) on D- (for delivery) Day by taking a hospital tour as your due date approaches.

Where you go depends on your hospital's policies and how you give birth. At many hospitals, you'll first go to a triage area, where a doctor or a nurse will check you and decide whether you're ready to be admitted to labor and delivery. At other institutions, if you arrive in labor, you'll be taken right to labor and delivery, where you'll change out of your street clothes and into a hospital gown. In some hospitals, you might spend your entire stay in the room in which you labor and deliver. In other hospitals, your postpartum room might even be on a different floor than labor and delivery, and you won't see it until you're wheeled there after giving birth. If you unexpectedly need a cesarean, you'll be taken from labor and delivery to an operating room devoted to the procedure. If you're having a scheduled cesarean, you might first go to the room in which you'll recuperate after delivery. Or, again, depending on your hospital, you might go directly to the operating suite where C-sections are performed.

Because of infection-control issues, it's unlikely that the operating rooms in which cesareans are performed will be part of your prenatal maternity unit tour, but you might get to see photographs of one in your childbirth preparation class. As you might expect, operating rooms are brightly lit and sterile-looking.

After your doctor examines you, you'll be asked to sign a consent form granting him permission to perform a cesarean (even if you're in labor and planning to deliver vaginally, you'll likely be asked to sign a C-section consent form, just in case). Hospital staff members will take your blood pressure, pulse, and temperature and listen to your baby's heartbeat. In most cases, they'll shave off a little of your pubic hair. To prepare for the remote possibility that you'll need general anesthesia, you also might be given medication to help dry your mouth and nose and reduce the acid in your stomach.

Shouldn't Hurt a Bit

An anesthesiologist will explain your options. In the not-so-good old days, doctors routinely knocked out women to deliver them, whether vaginally or by C-section.

Today, doctors put mothers to sleep only in extreme emergencies, when the baby must be delivered as quickly as possible by cesarean.

If your C-section is unplanned, you may have already received epidural anesthesia when you were in the labor and delivery room to relieve the pain of contractions.

This is how an epidural is administered: You'll be asked to curl up as much as possible, while you're on your side or seated on the edge of the bed. This opens the spaces between your vertebrae and allows the anesthesiologist to access the epidural space, which surrounds the membrane that contains the spinal fluid. The anesthesiologist will use a small needle to inject numbing medication into your skin. It might sting for a few seconds. Then she'll insert a very small plastic tube, or catheter, through your numb skin into the epidural space. A mixture of anesthesia and other painkillers will be injected into the catheter.

The drugs take effect in about 10 to 20 minutes. If you should later need a C-section, the anesthesiologist will inject additional anesthesia into the catheter to provide the higher level of numbness needed for the operation.

Looking Back

Obstetric anesthesia was first used in the United States to deliver a daughter to Fanny Longfellow, the wife of poet Henry Wadsworth Longfellow. The very next day, Henry visited Fanny's doctor, who also happened to be a dentist, to apprise him of his wife's condition and to have a tooth pulled . . . while anesthetized, of course.

If you're having a planned cesarean, or you need one after laboring without an epidural, you'll most likely get spinal anesthesia. The main difference between an epidural and a spinal is that the anesthetic and painkiller are injected right into the fluid that surrounds the spinal cord and connecting nerves, instead of into a tube leading to the epidural space. Spinal anesthesia works even more quickly than epidural anesthesia. One drawback with a spinal is a greater chance of a headache afterward. Perhaps 2 to 4 women out of 200 who get spinal anesthesia develop a headache afterward, compared to about 1 out of 200 who get an epidural.

With either an epidural or a spinal, your legs and abdomen should feel numb, but you'll remain awake. The most you should feel during a C-section is a slight tugging or pressure. If you feel more than that, tell a doctor or nurse immediately.

Susan M., 29, has had experience with both general anesthesia and epidurals, as well as emergency and planned C-sections. She delivered her firstborn by C-section under general anesthesia because the epidural she received didn't work quickly enough to allow immediate delivery of her baby. Preeclampsia had sent her blood pressure soaring, necessitating the emergency cesarean 10 weeks before

Looking Back

Cesarean section isn't named for Julius Caesar. Historians think the term cesarean (caesarean to the folks who prefer labour to labor and gynaecology to gynecology) stems from the Lex Caesare, or the Emperor's Law. That's because some other ancient Roman leader decreed that babies should be cut from the womb if their mothers died late in pregnancy. Other possible origins of the word cesarean include two Latin words: *caedare*, which means to cut, and *caesones*, which referred to babies delivered abdominally after their mothers had died.

her due date. Susan was pretty sick afterward, so she didn't get to hold her daughter, now 2 years old, until the next day. With her next baby, Susan opted for a planned cesarean with an epidural, scheduling it for the day before her due date. That way, the same doctor who had performed her first—and happened to be an old high school classmate—could do the honors.

"With the first C-section, I didn't know what was happening until it happened," she says. With her second, though, she had time to get nervous. She was concerned about being awake during surgery, but she needn't have worried. She didn't feel a thing, she says, but "I was there to witness my son's birth. I got to breastfeed him the day he was born. We bonded immediately, and I celebrated the fact that we had a healthy, full-term baby and an uneventful birth."

Before your doctor makes her first incision, you'll get a few more pokes in places other than where you get your epidural or spinal. A catheter will be inserted through your urethra and up into your bladder to drain urine during surgery, which is best performed on an empty bladder. (The opening to your urethra is located between your labia, below your clitoris and above your vagina.) If not already in place, a needle will be inserted into a vein in your hand or arm so you can receive fluids or, if necessary, medication during the operation. (Both will be removed about a day after your C-section.) Your belly will be washed with an antiseptic to reduce the chance of an infection. A blue surgical drape will be hung over your belly, blocking your view of the operation. You might have an oxygen mask placed over your mouth and nose to increase oxygen for your baby. You'll probably hear rustling and clanking as the nurses count the sponges and surgical instruments. Depending on your doctor and your wishes, your arms might be strapped down.

"What made it so wonderful was, number one, the labor

and delivery nurse. She was so incredibly fantastic," enthuses Annie, 35, who delivered her 5-month-old son by C-section because he was breech. "The second person—I sent him a thank-you note, he was so wonderful—was my anesthesiologist. He came in and introduced himself. He told me exactly what they were going to be doing. He made me relaxed by keeping me informed every step of the way. There was nothing that came as a surprise to me."

Once you're prepared for surgery, most hospitals will allow your husband or other designated person to enter the operating room and remain with you—unless there is an emergency that requires visitors to leave. A nurse will provide your partner with a set of ever-so-stylish scrub pants and shirt as well as a hat, mask, and shoe covers. Your support person can sit right next to you during the operation and hold your hand. But remember, no one is allowed to touch the sterile drapes that surround the surgical area and block your view of the proceedings. Some hospitals might allow your partner to photograph or tape the operation, while others ban taking pictures until afterward. Let your doctor know if you'd like to listen to favorite music brought from home.

Your doctor will make a low horizontal incision, or bikini cut (because it's so low a bikini will cover it), right across your pubic hair line, and then will cut or push aside fat and muscles to make an incision in your uterus. That 3- or 4-inch cut, like the exterior incision is usually horizontal and low, which results in less bleeding and a stronger scar than a vertical cut. However, depending on the position of your baby or placenta, you might need a vertical incision in your uterus.

After draining off the amniotic fluid, your doctor will gently pull your baby through your incisions. That's when you might hear your baby's first cry. You can ask that the surgical \drape be lowered so you can better see your doctor lift your baby out. Fluids are suctioned from the baby's mouth and nose, and the umbilical cord is clamped and cut. Your baby will then be handed to a nurse or, if necessary, a pediatrician who has been waiting in the operating room. Unless your baby needs to go to the nursery for special care (accompanied by your partner), she'll be washed and weighed and then handed to you. You can even start breastfeeding while your doctor is stitching you up. Ask for some help in finding a comfortable position and holding the baby.

At this point, you might be given antibiotics through your IV line to reduce the risk of an infection in your uterus or nearby organs, the most common complication of C-sections. Your doctor will then detach and remove the placenta and close the incision in your uterus with stitches that dissolve on their own. She'll use stitches or staples to close your abdomen.

"You feel pressure, and you're aware that people are pushing on you and working on you," recalls Dawn, 34, who chose to deliver her firstborn, now 13 months old, by cesarean, even though she could have delivered her vaginally. "You're lying on your back. You can't see anything that's going on because there is this big sheet blocking your view. It's really surreal."

TALKING POINT

If you want your partner to cut the cord after you have a C-section, tell your doctor ahead of time.

Looking Back

Up until the late 19th century, doctors were lucky that anyone survived a C-section. Besides their unsanitary working conditions, they omitted a critical step in the operation. In those days, all stitches had to be removed after a wound healed. It was impossible to remove stitches from the uterus after the abdomen had been closed, so doctors assumed that uterine contractions after delivery would control bleeding from the uterine incision. Wrong. Women often bled to death after a C-section, alleged to have the highest death rate of any surgical procedure at the time.

Max Sanger changed all that. In 1882, when he was 29 years old, the German gynecologist wrote a 200-page paper advocating that doctors close not only the incision in a patient's abdomen but also the one in her uterus. Sanger's persuasive argument really caught on. By the end of the 19th century, fewer than 10 percent of women died from delivering by cesarean.

Melanie, 28, delivered her daughter by a cesarean 5½ months ago. She had desperately wanted to have an unmedicated vaginal birth, but her baby turned into the breech position. She avoided having her arms strapped down on the operating table by promising she wouldn't move them.

As Melanie's doctor was about to lift the baby out of her uterus, she invited Melanie's husband, Ruffin, to peek over the surgical drape that had blocked the couple's view. Ruffin had served in the Marines for 6 years. He fought in Desert Storm. But nothing had prepared him for the sight of his wife's incision. When Melanie finally gave in to nausea, possibly a side effect from the morphine given with the anesthesia, Ruffin was asked to leave, "which I was more than happy to do then," he says. Ruffin now shares his experiences at a hospital "boot camp" for expectant fathers.

Although Ruffin might disagree, many women say they're pleasantly surprised about how quickly cesarean deliveries are accomplished. It takes only a few minutes to deliver the baby after an incision is made in the uterus. The whole operation, from when the first incision is made until it is completely sewn up, often takes less than an hour if no complications arise. Once it's over, you'll be taken to the recovery room, where you'll stay an hour or two, or as long as it takes for the epidural or spinal to wear off so that you can move your legs. (You'll most likely be in recovery longer if you've had general anesthesia.) If you're up to it, you can breastfeed your baby in the recovery room. (See "Close to the chest: Post-cesarean breast-feeding basics" on page 70).

When you're ready, a nurse will take you to the room where you'll spend the rest of your hospital stay, which typically lasts around 4 days—twice as long as for a vaginal delivery. Unless your baby needs special care, she should be able to stay with you the entire time, a set-up called "rooming-in." These days, few hospitals still require that all babies delivered by cesarean spend the first 24 hours of their lives under observation in the nursery, a separation that can greatly impede breastfeeding. If your hospital still has such a policy, ask your doctor to waive it

TALKING POINT

Restraining women's arms during a C-section is a rare practice these days, but if you're concerned about the prospect, talk to your doctor. If the hospital at which you are to deliver still insists upon restraints, ask that they strap down only the arm in which the IV line is inserted.

if your baby is healthy. If your baby has a health problem that prohibits her from rooming in, you should ask for a breast pump as soon as possible and pump every couple of hours. That will help stimulate your milk supply, and your baby can be fed the colostrum, or "foremilk," which comes in immediately after delivery.

GETTING THE BUGS OUT:
THE ROLE OF ANTIBIOTICS

That dose of antibiotics just after your C-section greatly reduces your chances of developing an infection in the lining of your uterus or your surgical wounds as a result of the operation. Cesarean delivery is the leading risk factor for such infections. Incisions make it that much easier for bugs that hang out harmlessly in your vagina to migrate into your womb. Postcesarean infections, signaled by a fever of 100.4 degrees or more, can lead to serious complications, even death. Yet, doctors routinely prescribe antibiotics to prevent infections only for women who've had unplanned C-sections. Concerns about cost and antibiotic resistance (that's when the drugs become ineffective due to overuse) have made doctors

Words from the Wise

Be aware that the antibiotics you're given after a C-section can occasionally cause thrush in your baby's mouth and on your nipples, possibly as early as a couple of weeks after birth. You may feel pain, itching, or burning on your nipples and you'll see white patches inside your baby's mouth and on her tongue and lips. She may or may not refuse to nurse. You'll both need to be treated, usually with an anti-fungal medication, to prevent you from re-infecting each other.

less eager to prescribe them for infection prevention in women undergoing scheduled cesareans.

The respected Cochrane Collaboration, an international nonprofit organization dedicated to spreading the scientific word about the effects of medical treatments, reviewed dozens of studies in which women undergoing C-sections were randomly assigned to receive antibiotics or have them withheld. Whether women delivered by planned or unplanned cesarean, antibiotics cut their risk of uterine infection by about 60 percent. Overall, the risk of wound infection was also reduced by about 60 percent, although the reduction was much greater in women who had unplanned C-sections.

THE PAIN OF IT ALL:
WHEN THE ANESTHESIA WEARS OFF

You don't have to suffer stoically like Andrea did after her C-section. If you had an epidural, chances are you received morphine as well as anesthesia through that tiny tube, or catheter, in your back. For about a day afterward, your doctor probably will leave the catheter in place to accommodate more doses of morphine. You might get a pump that allows you to control their timing.

Back in 1976, experiments in rats gave doctors the idea of administering morphine or other narcotic painkillers directly to the spines of patients after abdominal surgery. By taking that route, doctors could use far smaller doses of drugs than if they gave medications by mouth or intravenously, thus reducing side effects. Five years after scientists reported on their research with rats, the spinal approach to pain relief moved into obstetrics, enabling doctors to cut the required dose of narcotic painkillers by more than 95 percent in patients who've had a cesarean.

Narcotic painkillers aren't the only way to go, though. Some studies suggest that even the small doses delivered through the epidural catheter might make you somewhat more likely to experience side effects such as itchiness, nausea and vomiting, and slowed breathing. As an alternative, you might try ibuprofen, already a favorite for easing menstrual cramps (remember those?). Israeli researchers found that 400-milligram capsules of ibuprofen—the equivalent of two over-the-counter Advils or Motrins—provided satisfactory pain relief after C-sections, with no serious side effects and with no need for equipment that could restrict your access to your baby, such as a catheter in your spine and an IV pole. Many hospitals now combine the best of both worlds by giving patients ibuprofen or other non-steroidal anti-inflammatory drugs (NSAIDs), such as naproxen by mouth, along with very low doses of narcotic painkillers in the spine.

In the Israeli study, women who received the ibuprofen at fixed times during the day were more satisfied than women who received the medication only when they asked for it. That just goes to show you: There's no point in waiting until you can't stand the pain anymore before requesting more medication. Ask for it even before you need it, advises Sue, because if you wait, you might not get it before your previous dose wears off.

Even if you're connected to a morphine drip, you can—and should—get

> **Words from the Wise**
>
> *Ibuprofen often can provide adequate post-cesarean pain relief without the side effects sometimes seen with morphine. Don't be a martyr, though. Keep ahead of your pain by asking for medication before you feel the need for it.*

out of bed and walk, if only to the bathroom. (You might find it difficult to urinate the first day or so, due to the effect of anesthesia on your bladder). Walking might be the furthest thing from your mind, but it can actually help

Words from the Wise

If you feel a cough, laugh, or sneeze coming on, hold a pillow against your incision to support it.

relieve the pain and prevent the formation of blood clots in deep veins, a very rare but dangerous complication of C-sections. "I think the biggest thing is to get up and get moving as soon as you can after the surgery. If it takes pain medication to do that, fine," says Beth, 36, who delivered her firstborn, now age 6½, vaginally and her second, age 5, unexpectedly by C-section. She plans to deliver her third by a repeat cesarean. "Tolerate a little pain. It's not the end of the world. I wouldn't be afraid of it."

Lisa's mom is a surgical nurse, so she knows how important it is not to lie around after an operation. "She's also not the most pampering person," Lisa says. The day after 34-year-old Lisa delivered her son, now age 3, her mom had her walking the hospital halls holding a pillow over her stomach for support. In a pinch, as Lisa learned from her mom, you can use a pillow to support your incision when you cough, laugh, or sneeze.

After Kathryn delivered her eighth baby, the fourth of her five cesarean deliveries, her doctor prescribed a special wrap-around girdle that literally girded her against pain from her incision. (Once you're home from the hospital, some women recommend wearing tight bicycle shorts under your clothes for the same reason.) "It felt great," Kathryn says. "I was religious about it." She wore that girdle day and night, even for a few days after she got home.

FINE DINING:
NO REASON TO STARVE AFTER A C-SECTION

Go ahead and have lunch (or breakfast or dinner) after your C-section if you feel like it. The longstanding tradition of withholding food and drink after surgery—have to let the gut settle down after all that anesthesia and trauma, you know—appears to be unwarranted in women who have just had cesareans. Most C-sections are performed under regional, not general, anesthesia and require little handling of the intestines, so they might not disrupt bowel function at all. In fact, some research suggests that eating soon after a cesarean delivery might actually speed your recovery.

Policies about food and drink after C-sections vary widely. Some doctors and hospitals let women eat and drink within a few hours of a cesarean, while others ban anything by mouth for 24 hours or more. Not to be indelicate about it, but basically many doctors and hospitals withhold food until you pass gas, a sign that your gut is up and running after surgery.

Now the doctors and nurses pretty much have to take your word on this one, so you might just want to let the rumble of your stomach, not your intestines, dictate when you dine. Not long after her first C-section, Sue remembers visiting a friend who had

Words from the Wise

Some doctors and hospitals won't let you eat or drink for 24 hours or more after a C-section. They want to make sure your post-op gut is up to handling it, as demonstrated by your ability to pass gas. But if you feel like eating before that first "toot," just say you did and ask for a menu. If you have gas pains after surgery, it's probably best to avoid food, such as beans, or drinks—too hot, too cold, or carbonated—that could exacerbate them.

just had one. "She had a midwife who told her, 'Just lie to them. They want you to pass gas before you eat. If you feel like you're ready to eat, tell them you passed gas.'"

Cheryl's firstborn is now 16, but she still remembers the hunger pangs that gnawed at her after he was delivered by an unplanned cesarean. "No one fed me for 2 days after the baby was born. By the time they did, I told them, 'I'm kind of really happy.'" For the first 24 hours after each of her five C-sections, Kathryn wasn't supposed to drink water, let alone eat. All she was allowed was ice chips. Fortunately, she was more tired than hungry, but there was no way that ice chips could quench the thirst she always felt after the operation. She drank water before getting her doctor's okay and the main thing that happened was she didn't feel so thirsty anymore. (In addition, drinking lots of water and cranberry juice after a cesarean can minimize your chances of developing a urinary tract infection from the catheter that had been inserted into your bladder.)

Discrepancies in hospital policies about food and drink after cesarean deliveries spurred the Cochrane Collaboration to examine the scientific evidence behind them. The group reviewed six studies in which women were randomly assigned to receive food and drink relatively early—usually within 6 to 8 hours of surgery—or much later. It concluded that the studies' findings did not justify denying food and drink to hungry or thirsty patients who need all their strength to recover from C-sections as well as to care for their newborns.

Eating relatively soon after a C-section could shorten your hospital stay, suggests a study from CHRISTUS St. Joseph Hospital in Houston. Researchers there randomly divided willing patients into two groups. One was allowed to eat regular food within 4 to 8 hours of undergoing a C-section, while the other was allowed nothing by mouth for 12 to 24 hours afterward, and then received only clear liquids on the first post-op day. That group had to wait a couple of days for solid food. The women who ate early—on average, 5 hours after their C-section—were no more likely to develop gas pains (a common occurrence after abdominal surgery) than those who ate late. In fact, the early eaters had a bowel movement sooner than the late eaters (that's a good thing) and, on average, left the hospital just 2 full days after delivery, compared to 3 full days for the late eaters.

NOT MISSING THE BLOAT: BUBBLES YOU'LL WANT TO BURST

Forget about your abdomen (if you can). Immediately after a C-section, you might feel even more pain in your shoulders. Don't worry, your obstetrician didn't slip while making an incision in your abdomen. In fact, the pain isn't even coming from your shoulders. What you're experiencing is called referred pain, which simply means it originated in another part of your body—which brings us back to your abdomen. During any abdominal surgery, gas can get trapped there or in your intestines. The good news is that it will go away before you leave the hospital. The bad news is that it can really hurt until then. "I felt like there was an elephant sitting on my chest," recalls Dawn.

But there are steps you can take to get rid of trapped gas. You've heard this before: Walk, walk, walk. If you're not up to walking down the hall, at least walk around your room. You'll feel better for it. Really. By the day after she underwent her second unplanned C-section, Jaime was walking to the nursery to get her daughter. She never stopped walking in the hospital unless she was tired or in a lot of pain, and she believes this really helped her "get the gas out quicker."

When you rest after all that exercise, do it in a rocking chair if possible. That back-and-forth motion helps push the gas out. Avoid drinking beverages that are very hot, very cold, or carbonated, all of which can increase gassiness, as can drinking through a straw. For that matter, avoid gassy foods, although it's unlikely the hospital cafeteria is going to whip up wieners and beans and sauerkraut for dinner.

A nurse might give you an over-the-counter medication that contains simethicone, such as Gas-X or Mylanta Gas. Simethicone isn't absorbed by the body, so it's okay to take while breastfeeding, but studies have found it no more effective than a sugar pill. Couldn't hurt, though.

Or you might prefer to try a folk remedy. Some women swear by peppermint or ginger tea. For Anita, m-o-l-a-s-s-e-s spelled relief. "Though no doctor would admit that I was a likely candidate for a C-section, being a fairly small woman gave me a suspicion. So while I went through all the motions of learning Lamaze, I quietly collected wisdom on C-sections. The best piece of information came from a nurse who admitted right up front that she had no idea why this worked, but it did—not only for C-sections but for other abdominal surgery. Take 1 tablespoon of molasses in a cup of hot water—molasses tea, in effect—and drink a cup three times a day to prevent gas pains." When Anita packed her bag for the hospital, she included a bottle of dark molasses and a tablespoon, just in case. Turns out her intuition served her well. She did indeed end up with a C-section but no gas pains,

Words from the Wise

Got gas? Take a hike, then relax by rocking in a rocking chair and sip molasses or peppermint tea (not too hot, though). Some women swear by these folk remedies.

thanks, she's sure, to the molasses. "Four years later, I repeated it with my second daughter with the same success. By then, I'd also learned that molasses was a good source of iron—a bonus for blood-building."

Anita's daughters are in graduate school and college now, but their mother is still proselytizing about the miracle of molasses. Whenever she visits a friend who's just had abdominal surgery, a cesarean or otherwise, she comes bearing a bottle and a tablespoon. "The brave take it and have had great results. The trick is to let it be the first thing in your digestive tract as it gets back to work. I quite like the taste, though I know it's not everyone's cup of tea, so to speak." To make molasses more palatable, try mixing a tablespoon with tea, juice, or milk three times a day.

CLOSE TO THE CHEST: POST-CESAREAN BREASTFEEDING BASICS

Just because you have a C-section doesn't mean you can't try to breastfeed right away. Besides providing optimal nutrition for your baby, breastfeeding helps your uterus shrink to its normal, pre-pregnancy size. You'll even feel it contract while you nurse, a sensation called "after pain." However, some research suggests that if you deliver by C-section, it may take a little longer for your milk to come in than if you'd delivered vaginally. That's due partly to how you might be feeling and partly to how your baby might be feeling. You might need a little extra time before you're up to holding and nursing the baby. Meanwhile, your baby might be a little drowsy and lethargic from your anesthesia, so she might not latch on enthusiastically right away. But don't worry about how the painkillers you're taking might affect your baby. Although the drugs are found in breast milk, they're generally

TALKING POINT

Make sure that you let your doctor know if you'd like to breastfeed your baby right after delivering by C-section. You might be able to start nursing right on the operating table while your doctor finishes stitching you up. Remember, the sooner you start, the sooner your mature milk will come in.

harmless to you and your baby, who just might get a little sleepy from them.

If you want to hold your baby and try to breastfeed as soon as possible after the birth, make sure you tell your doctor beforehand. Your husband, nurse, or doula can prop you up a little and help you to position and support your baby.

If you can't find a comfortable position, ask your doctor or nurse to get you help from a lactation consultant who's experienced in working with women who've had a C-section. You might not want to hold your baby across your abdomen in the traditional cradle hold when you breastfeed. Many women prefer the football hold, which kind of looks like it sounds. The baby is tucked to one side of you, under your arm and supported by pillows, while your hand holds the base of her head and neck. Or, at first, you might feel most comfortable lying down on your side, tummy-to-tummy with your baby. After a day or two, when you're feeling a little better, you might prefer the cradle hold. Simply put a pillow over your abdomen and your baby on top of the pillow.

Breastfeeding was a priority for Melanie, even though she didn't always "feel so hot."

"Sometimes it would have been a lot easier just to give her a bottle," she says. "If breastfeeding's not important to you, that's fine. But it was very important to me."

Ellen says she would have rather used her brief time in the hospital to recuperate from surgery. "I think they really pressure you to take care of the baby all night. When you've just had a baby, maybe you could use the sleep overnight," says Ellen. "I don't think anyone can prove to me that if babies miss one or two feedings in the middle of the night, they're not going to breastfeed."

If you're looking for another reason to try breastfeeding, consider this: Research in mice suggests it could help hasten the healing of your surgical wounds. Ohio State University researchers studied mice that were nursing their pups (yup, that's what they call baby mice) and mice that were not nursing, either because their pups had been taken away or because they had never mated. The scientists gave all of the mice a superficial skin wound on the scruff of their neck. Each day for 12 days, the researchers measured the size of the

TALKING POINT

Ask a hospital lactation consultant to help you find comfortable positions for breastfeeding after a C-section. At first, you might find nursing while lying on your side most comfortable; but after a little while, you might prefer the traditional cradle hold, with the baby resting on a pillow over your abdomen.

wounds to determine how quickly they were healing. The nursing mice healed significantly faster than the never-mated mice. The researchers found that in mice, at least, lactation suppresses

Words from the Wise

Breastfeeding actually might help your incision to heal more quickly.

stress hormones and alters immune function, leading to speedier wound healing. Believe it or not, they say that rodents and women undergo similar hormonal changes after birth and while nursing, so what's good for the mouse might also be good for the mother. The scientists next plan to compare wound healing in new moms who choose to breastfeed versus those who opt for bottle-feeding.

CHAPTER 3

RECOVERING QUICKLY

Strategies to ease pain
and speed healing

This is a tale of two C-sections. They were both Sue's, but her recovery from each was about as different as possible. Sue, 36, delivered her first daughter by cesarean about 2 months early. Sue went home four days afterward, but her daughter had to stay in the intensive care nursery for 7 weeks until she put on a little weight. The separation was tough, although Sue was able to breastfeed her daughter. She listened to her doctor and didn't drive for a few weeks, so her husband chauffeured her to see their daughter. The baby was doing fine, giving Sue plenty of time to rest after surgery. "I didn't have a baby at home. I wasn't waking up in the middle of the night," she says.

Less than 2 years later, Sue was on the operating table to deliver daughter number two by a planned cesarean a week before her due date. The operation went more smoothly, and she was ready to go home more quickly than after her first delivery. She had the baby on Tuesday, and they both went home on Thursday, even though her doctor would have preferred that they both stay another day. "My OB/GYN didn't want me to go home. Because of the other baby, she knew that I would probably not get a good night's sleep." But

Sue figured anything had to be better than the hospital. "You just don't sleep well in the hospital. They're vacuuming the hallway at 2 o'clock in the morning."

Sleep was the least of her concerns. Sue now had a baby and a toddler to care for, as well as her post-cesarean self. Her parents came to help out for the first 2 weeks. By the time they left, Sue's doctor told her she could drive. But there was another doctor's order that Sue could not obey. No way. "I wasn't supposed to lift the 22-month-old for a month. That, of course, didn't happen. What was I supposed to do? She was still in a crib."

MOTHERING THE NEW MOM: CARING FOR YOURSELF WHILE YOU CARE FOR YOUR BABY

You just had major surgery, your hormones are raging and on top of everything else, you have a newborn to take care of. Welcome to motherhood.

While this advice really goes for any woman who's just had a baby, it's especially important for any woman who's just had a baby via a C-section:

- Don't hesitate to accept help, whether it's your husband volunteering to change diapers or a neighbor offering to cook dinner.
- Sleep, or at least rest, whenever the baby does.
- If you can afford it, consider hiring a postpartum doula to help you out around the house.
- Don't beat yourself up for not feeling your happiest, most energetic best. That time will come, probably sooner than you expect.

As a rule of thumb, it usually takes about 6 weeks for women to feel more like their pre-pregnancy selves after having a C-section. For much of that time, you'll have a vaginal discharge (the leftover gunk in your uterus has to get out somehow) called lochia, which is bright red at first and then gradually changes to yellow or white. It may last up to 4 weeks, so stock up on sanitary pads, because you shouldn't use tampons for the first 6 weeks after delivery.

Even if you feel better fairly quickly after your C-section, don't go overboard and try to do too much. That can be tough when you have other children and no help during the day, but doctors generally have good reasons for their post-cesarean instructions. Take the ban on driving. In the first week or two after you give birth, sleep deprivation and/or pain medication can impair your reflexes. If you feel up to driving, have someone ride shotgun with you to make sure you're really ready. If you notice your copilot sitting with eyes squeezed shut or hands clasped tight in prayer, better wait another week or two before driving solo.

Words from the Wise

Stock up on maxi-pads before you leave for the hospital. Whether you deliver vaginally or by C-section, you'll have a vaginal discharge for up to 4 weeks after you give birth. And you're not supposed to use tampons until your baby is 6 weeks old.

If you ask Juliet, recovery from a C-section gets easier with practice. She delivered all three of her daughters by C-section, and at age 38, she was already a "geriatric mother"—gotta love those terms—when she gave birth to her first. Despite her increasing age—she was 46 when her third daughter was born 2 years ago—Juliet says recovery became easier with each birth. "My body learned to heal better and better after each one. After my first cesarean, I couldn't walk up and down the stairs. I couldn't cough." By the time her third daughter was born, "I was literally up and walking around at the end of that day. We actually drove to Maine for our summer vacation 5 days later." She just had to make sure to stop every hour and a half so she could get out of the car and walk around to minimize the post-surgery risk of blood clots deep in her veins.

> **Words from the Wise**
>
> *Common sense rules the road when it comes to driving. If you can barely keep your eyes open, if you're still taking heavy-duty painkillers or if you're having trouble focusing on anything but your baby (and who could blame you?), do yourself, your family, and society at large a favor and ride on the passenger side for awhile.*

Don't worry if you're not up to traveling the week (or month) after your cesarean. In fact, don't worry if you're not up to doing much of anything at first. "I think the prevailing wisdom is that the wife will be able to take care of the baby when she gets home from the hospital," says Ruffin, whose wife, Melanie, delivered their firstborn by C-section because the baby was breech. "Even with a vaginal delivery, from what I understand, it's really hard to do that for the first few days. Melanie was on Percocet for 3 weeks. She was incapacitated for the most part, except for breastfeeding."

The problem is, Ruffin had never taken Baby Care 101, let alone more advanced training. "I was not prepared to take 100 percent full care of the baby," to put it mildly. But the former Marine is one resourceful guy. "I flagged the nurse down in the recovery room and told her I'd certainly never, ever changed a diaper, and I'd never seen a baby girl. She said, 'I'm glad you asked' and was very methodical about it."

Once Melanie left the hospital, 3 days after her daughter's birth, "I changed pretty much every diaper for the first 3 weeks or so," Ruffin says. He knows he was lucky to have been able to afford to take that much time off from his work in real estate.

Sometimes, not even moms can afford to take time off from their work after having a C-section. Ellen, 42, who's now a family practice doctor, was near the end of her second year of medical school when she delivered her first baby by cesarean. "You decide what you want to do and what's important. I wanted to get through medical school." A week after her daughter's birth, Ellen boarded a commuter train from her suburban home and headed back to medical school to take a test. The test involved examining a patient and taking his medical history, as her professor looked on. "I wasn't thrilled about that, but it beat the alternative," she says. If she hadn't joined her class on the day the test was scheduled, she would have had to take it alone, her professor's center of attention.

Isabel, 42, was 6 months pregnant with her first daughter, now age 5, when she interviewed for a job. The company overlooked her condition and hired her. "I'm not going to let you down," she told her boss. "I'll go right back

Words from the Wise

It's probably best to wait at least a month before going on a trip that will require you to sit for an extended period of time. If you must travel, though, make sure to get up and walk around every hour or so to keep the blood circulating in your legs. That will reduce your risk of developing blood clots, a rare but serious complication of surgery.

to work." A single mother, she basically had no maternity leave with daughter number one, who was delivered by an unplanned C-section. "The day I had the baby was a Friday. I was home by Sunday. And on Monday morning I was on the phones again making calls and working." She probably couldn't have done it without the help of a nanny 5

> ## Words from the Wise
>
> *Baby-care classes are not just for expectant moms. First-time dads-to-be should also take the opportunity to learn the basics of diapering and bathing. And if dad can take off work for the first couple of weeks after the baby comes home, all the better.*

days a week. Three months after her daughter's birth, Isabel was back in the office, bringing an end to breastfeeding. Her employer wasn't as understanding when she got pregnant again about 2 years later. Isabel got fired and settled a lawsuit against the company out of court. After her second daughter was born, Isabel had no job to rush back to. It took much of her life savings, but she spent a year not working. "I just came back and breastfed that baby."

THE KINDEST CUT: TAKING CARE OF YOUR INCISION

When asked in a recent survey what the most uncomfortable part of their C-section was, mothers who'd delivered less than 2 years earlier cited pain from their incision, which is not exactly surprising. Some said the pain persisted for 6 months. While your incision might hurt, you'll feel numbness above it because nerves in your skin were cut during surgery. Normal sensation should return by the time your baby is a year old.

Meanwhile, chances are you'll feel most of the usual aches and pains of new mothers, such as mild uterine cramping, especially if you're breastfeeding and it's not your first baby. But just think—you won't have to deal with a sore perineum, that little area between the thighs that gets quite a workout, if not cut and stitched, during a vaginal delivery. Perhaps you've had the experience of having to sit on one of those donut-shaped pillows after delivering vaginally. "With a vaginal delivery, it was pain in a different place," recalls Kathryn. "I had that episiotomy, and that was sore."

Your doctor's ban on heavy lifting—that is, anything heavier than your baby—is meant to prevent you from injuring your incision and ending up with a hernia. For similar reasons, your doctor also will tell you to use a stepstool instead of stretching to reach a high shelf and to keep stair-climbing to a minimum. For a while after her C-section, 34-year-old Dawn found she needed a stepstool to get into her bed at home.

Also, sit on firm, straight-backed chairs. Think of the strain on your abdomen when you get up out of a soft chair, especially one in which you sink so much that your bottom is lower than your knees. When you were 8 or

Words from the Wise

Take off from work for as long as possible after your baby is born. If you have a C-section, you're going to need a little extra recovery time than if you deliver vaginally. Don't wait until the last minute to arrange your maternity leave with your employer. There will be paperwork to fill out and plans to be made about who will handle your responsibilities while you're out. And don't kid yourself about getting a lot of work done from home while you're away from the office. Unless you have full-time help, babies have a knack for interrupting phone calls and trains of thought. But you probably wouldn't have it any other way.

9 months pregnant, you might have even needed your husband to pull you up out of your cushiest chair. Compare that to how you can practically pop up out of firm, straight-backed chair, maybe like the ones around your dining room table.

A small proportion of C-section patients develop an infection in their incision, so it's important to keep yours clean and dry. You can shower or take a bath as long as the edges of your incision aren't open. If you have those little white pieces of tape on your incision, feel free to pull them off once you get home (if they haven't already fallen off in the shower or tub). It's normal to see a little pink, watery fluid draining from the incision, but you should call your doctor if any of the following happens:

● The drainage begins to smell bad
● Your incision is more tender, or redder than usual, or swollen
● The edges of the incision separate
● You run a fever over 100.4 degrees

> **Words from the Wise**
>
> *Make sure you have a stepstool in your kitchen so you don't have to stretch your tender abdomen when reaching for something on a top shelf. If you have one of those high pillow-top mattresses on your bed, keep another stepstool next to it to avoid stretching when you get in and out.*

TALKING POINT

Call your doctor if your incision doesn't seem to be healing properly. That could be a sign of an infection.

Any of these might be a symptom of an infection that requires treatment with antibiotics.

Cynthia, who delivered her 3-month-old twins by cesarean, not only kept her eyes closed during the operation but refused to look at her incision for 3 months afterward. "I'm pretty queasy about things like this," she explains. "I would just have my husband look at it to make sure it was healing properly." When she finally did take a peek, though, "it wasn't so bad."

The last of Janice's three C-sections was 14 years ago, but her scar can still be tender. "Isn't that weird? Just on the ends of it, not through the middle," says Janice, 49. After her incision had completely closed and healed, Janice used to break open capsules of vitamin E and rub it on her scar to minimize its appearance. Many doctors recommend trying vitamin E for that purpose, but studies of its effectiveness have had mixed results.

Sex might be the least of your concerns right now, which is probably a good thing. Most doctors advise not having sex for at least 6 weeks after delivery, whether or not you've had a C-section. If you've had a C-section, you want to your incision to be well on the way to being healed before you strain it or put pressure on it during sex, or else you might be setting yourself up for a uterine infection, which is not a fun thing.

> **Words from the Wise**
>
> *You might feel like having sex sooner, but wait until your baby is at least 6 weeks old. You have some healing to do first. And remember, even if you're breastfeeding and even if your periods haven't resumed yet, you can still get pregnant, so talk to your doctor about birth control. (Your pre-pregnancy diaphragm won't fit properly anymore, you know.)*

This is especially important to remember if you have a particularly, ahem, energetic partner.

If you were in labor and your cervix was starting to dilate before you had a C-section, you have another

Words from the Wise

You might experience vaginal dryness, especially if you're breastfeeding. A lubricant can help.

reason to wait at least 6 weeks before you have sex. That's about the time your cervix will have closed. Until then, your open cervix, plus all the blood and gunk coming out of your uterus, further increases your risk of developing a uterine infection if you have sex.

SHAPING UP:
HOW AND WHEN TO EXERCISE
AFTER A C-SECTION

You probably won't feel like returning to your spinning class when you get home from the hospital, and you shouldn't. Walking is a must to prevent blood clots and decrease muscle stiffness, but take it easy at first. Aerobic exercise should wait until your baby is about 6 weeks old, but you can start pelvic floor-tightening exercises within a few days of delivery.

Even though you had a C-section, your risk of eventually developing pelvic floor problems, such as incontinence, is still higher than that of a woman who's never been pregnant. If you've never done Kegel exercises, now would be a good time to start. Simply tighten the muscles around your vagina, as if you were stopping a urine stream, and your rectum, as if you were stopping a bowel movement. Hold for a few seconds, relax, then repeat.

To help strengthen your abdomen, try pelvic tilts a couple weeks after delivery. Simply get on your hands and knees and pull in your stomach to arch your back. Hold for 3 to 5 seconds and then repeat five to 10 times. Crunches will have to wait until your doctor gives you the go-ahead, which usually is around that magic 6-week mark. (Sex and exercise do have a lot in common, you know.) If, like some women, your abdominal muscles separated as your pregnant belly expanded (a condition called diastasis recti), you'll have to wait a couple of weeks longer before you start doing crunches.

Melanie was a runner before she got pregnant, and she continued to run on and off until she was about 4 months along. After her C-section, she figured she certainly was in good enough shape to accomplish a routine household task. She soon realized her mistake. "When I first got home, I thought maybe I'll just do laundry from the hospital. But I couldn't even bend over to get things out of the dryer." So she started slowly working toward her goal of running again. "My first exercise was to the end of my road and back," says Melanie, who lives on a cul-de-sac. "Then I would walk around the block. I just kept trying to exercise a little bit every day. It was whatever I felt comfortable doing."

Sue resumed working out more quickly after her second cesarean than after her first. But then, her deliveries were under such dif-

Words from the Wise

Even if you deliver by C-section, simply being pregnant can increase your risk of developing incontinence later in life. Kegel exercises can help tighten your pelvic floor muscles, and you can do them anywhere—no special equipment needed.

ferent circumstances. With her first pregnancy, Sue developed a rare condition that caused her blood pressure to shoot up, among other things. Because her baby was premature, Sue was reluctant to put her in the care of the babysitter at the Y. But she was fine during her second pregnancy. "I was playing tennis until a couple days

Words from the Wise

Even if you ran marathons before you got pregnant, resume your exercise program gradually after you deliver. By the time your baby is 6 weeks old, you'll be ready to return to running or other aerobic exercises.

before the baby arrived." And exactly 6 weeks after giving birth, Sue was back at the Y, her toddler and her baby in the facility's nursery. She still hasn't gone back to playing tennis, although she's certainly up for it. "It's just too hard with the two of them."

EMOTIONAL BAGGAGE?
THE PSYCHOLOGICAL IMPACT
OF HAVING A CESAREAN

A few studies in the early and mid-1990s suggested that women were more likely to suffer postpartum depression after a C-section than after a vaginal birth. But more recent research has found no connection between mode of delivery and risk of postpartum depression.

However, individual women's reactions to having a cesarean vary widely. Some use words like failure, guilt, grief, and mourning to describe their feelings. They feel like they missed out on a fundamental life experience by not delivering vaginally. Yet, other women credit their C-section for their baby's safe arrival. They view delivery as a means to an end, nothing more.

Jaime readily acknowledges that she suffered from depression after delivering her first daughter, now about a year old, by an unplanned cesarean. "You build yourself up for that big moment when your baby comes out. When I didn't get that, and I was just laid up on a cold table with my arms spread and a drape over me, and I didn't get to see the baby come out, I literally felt I failed. It was just an overwhelming sadness."

Megan's emotional recovery from her C-section lasted far longer than the physical. "I was very angry for over a year. I never went back to that doctor for a checkup." She skipped the standard 2-week post-cesarean checkup altogether. For her 6-week postpartum checkup, she saw a nurse practitioner at the hospital where she worked. Her sense of failure lingered. "I was disappointed that I didn't stand up for myself more. I could have been stronger at that point." To help overcome her negative feelings, Megan underwent a few sessions of what she describes as "birth trauma counseling." Her counselor suggested that she stop thinking of her son's delivery as an operation. "Instead of calling it a cesarean section, she ended up calling it a cesarean birth. That was an incredible part of my healing process."

Anne can't imagine what it's like to have a vaginal de-

> **Words from the Wise**
>
> *Even if you don't have a sitter, you can find time to exercise. Check with local hospitals for "Mommy and Me" exercise classes, which are also a great way to meet other new moms. See whether the Y or any health clubs offer child care while you work out. If the weather's nice, go for a hike with your baby. If it's not, get moving with an exercise video. She'll like the music.*

livery. At age 44, she's had three C-sections. The first was performed because her son, now 19, was breech. The vertical incision in her uterus necessitated that her second and third sons, now 16 and 14, also be delivered by cesarean. "I felt like I was so robbed, especially after I found out I could never have a vaginal delivery," she says.

Words from the Wise

If you're feeling down because you didn't have the birth you'd planned on, call the hospital where you delivered to see whether it has a support group for moms who had C-sections. Or ask if there's a social worker you can talk to.

"You have to work through it. It's like a grieving process, really." To deal with her disappointment, Anne focused on her doctor's advice: "It's not how you have them, it's how you raise them."

Sure, "there's a lot of shocking things about a C-section," says Susan M., 29, who's had two, the first an emergency because of preeclampsia, the second planned. "Okay, you didn't have the birth you wanted, and then you're put back together with staples. It's so freaky you can't believe it's your own body." But Susan shakes her head when she hears women talk about having failed because they had a C-section instead of a vaginal delivery. She thinks they'd be better off if they focused on their baby's well-being, rather than their own notion of an ideal delivery. That's just one example of how motherhood has a way of rearranging women's priorities.

Still, it's not unusual for women to blame themselves for not having their ideal birth, notes childbirth educator Carol Wyman of Fairfax, Virginia. They assume they must not have exercised enough or eaten the right foods. If you still feel that way a few months after your baby is born, Wyman advises, you might

Words from the Wise

If you feel the need to talk with other women who've had C-sections but find it inconvenient to attend support group meetings, simply log on to your computer. A number of Web sites and newsgroups offer the opportunity for new mothers to chat online—especially comforting when you can't fall back to sleep after a 2:00 A.M. feeding. (See Resources, page 197, for information about how to connect with them.)

want to follow Megan's example and seek counseling. A support group or class for women who've had a cesarean can also be helpful, she says.

Take care of yourself, enjoy your baby, and don't let anyone make you feel bad about having had a C-section. All too quickly, your delivery will be ancient history—sigh—and you'll be focusing on preschool picks and potty training.

PART 2

Making the Decision: Yes or No?

CHAPTER 4

A MATTER OF CHOICE

When you want to ask for a C-Section

Clair, 43, can quickly list several reasons for choosing to deliver her 9-week-old daughter via C-section. None of them are medical.

"I knew it would be less stress for me," she says. "I'm a single mom. The only thing that concerned me throughout the entire pregnancy was what if my water breaks and I'm alone? I talked to my doctor about it, and it clearly would be less stress on the baby."

Her fertility specialist and her OB/GYN assured her that there was no evidence to suggest that babies delivered vaginally were healthier than those delivered by cesarean. In other words, Clair was told there was no medical reason not to have a C-section.

By scheduling the C-section, Clair could plan accordingly, both professionally and personally. She runs her own company, and her parents live out of town, and they're older. Knowing exactly when she was going to deliver was a plus, if not a must.

And finally, Clair thought, a planned cesarean delivery would leave nothing to chance medically. "If I could not be in control of the situation, then I wanted my doctor to be in

*control," she says. "I love my doctor. A friend of mine calls
me the poster girl for C-sections. It's not right for everyone,
but it was absolutely the right thing for me."*

If you can choose to get breast implants or a tummy tuck,
you should be able to opt for a C-section over a vaginal delivery,
right? That's the argument put forth by a small but growing number
of women—reportedly including celebrities Claudia Schiffer, Elizabeth Hurley, and Victoria "Posh Spice" Beckham—who know from
the outset, sometimes even before they conceive, that they want a cesarean. British headline writers describe them as "too posh to push."

Dawn James is neither supermodel nor singer, but she em-
pathizes with fellow Brits Hurley and Beckham. "There is this
group of women who have this attitude that it is macho to go
through the pain of childbirth," James, 37, a management consultant, told a London newspaper 3 months after delivering her son by
C-section for no reason other than the fact that she wanted to do
it that way. "Why should I have to do that? I would not walk the
streets of London with a screaming headache and not take a
painkiller. I feel very strongly that people or organizations who seek
to make women feel guilty about not going through childbirth in
a natural manner are evil."

Rebecca Eckler, a columnist for the *National Post* newspaper
in Canada, acknowledged that her decision to have a planned cesarean for no medical reason was controversial. "I had told only a
few people I already knew the date—October 15—that baby
Rowan would be born, after realizing people have stronger views
on C-sects than they do on religion or politics," Eckler wrote just
a week after her daughter's birth. "You cannot do a C-sect," one
of her friends who'd already gone the mommy route told her, "unless you have to. You won't be able to pick up your baby for weeks.
It's very painful and can be dangerous for you and the baby. Be a

hero and do it the vaginal way." I am no hero, I told her, and changed the subject immediately.

Perhaps you're of like mind. Chances are you could deliver vaginally if you wanted to. Maybe you al-

> ## Words from the Wise
>
> *C-sections, especially if they're planned, are much safer today than they were when you were born.*

ready have. You're healthy, you've never had a cesarean and you're carrying only one baby and it's not breech—in other words, there's no compelling medical reason for you to schedule a C-section. In fact, doctors would say you're at a low risk of needing a cesarean if you were to go into labor. No matter. C-sections are safer than ever, so you figure that the benefits of the procedure might now actually outweigh the risks.

You'd rather schedule a C-section than take the chance you'd end up having one anyway after hours and hours of labor. You've heard that C-sections are safer than vaginal deliveries for babies and less likely to lead to incontinence and other "female problems." You can't understand why some women make such a big deal out of the experience of giving birth vaginally. Maybe you're anxious about the pain and uncertainty of labor. And you have to admit that the thought of being able to schedule your baby's birth—ensuring that the nursery will be ready and the grandparents standing by—adds to the appeal of a cesarean. Before you make up your mind about whether to request a C-section, let's take a look at the advantages and drawbacks.

TAKING CONTROL: THE GROWING TREND OF PATIENT-CHOICE C-SECTIONS

Although patient-choice C-sections are only a small fraction of the million or so cesareans performed in the U.S. each year, there are signs that they're increasing in the United States and elsewhere. At the very least, they appear to be attracting more attention:

- The most recent annual meeting of the Society for Maternal-Fetal Medicine, a professional group of OB/GYNs, featured a roundtable discussion of the question: "Is vaginal delivery obsolete?"

- A recent nationwide survey of 1,600 women who had given birth within the previous 2 years included a question about whether they would choose a cesarean next time. While 71 percent said "not likely at all," and another 12 percent said "not very likely," the fact that the survey even asked the question is noteworthy.

- A study of hospital discharge data by HealthGrades, a Denver consulting firm that evaluates healthcare quality, suggests that about 63,000 U.S. women opted for a C-section in 2001 even though there was no pressing medical reason for them to have one. That represented a 20 percent increase over 1999, although it was still a small proportion of deliveries.

W. Benson Harer, M.D., a past president of the American College of Obstetricians and Gynecologists, thinks there were probably even more patient-choice C-sections than HealthGrades found. To avoid opening themselves up to questions about the medical necessity of such deliveries, doctors usually come up with reasons for doing them, says Harer, medical director of Riverside County Regional Medical Center in Moreno Valley, California. Macrosomia (when a newborn weighs 8 pounds, 12 ounces or more) is a handy excuse, because accurately predicting a baby's birth weight before delivery is virtually impossible. "We can't estimate the sizes of babies at all," says Harer, who helped spur the ongoing national debate about patient-choice cesareans. "If it looks at all iffy, then we go with macrosomia."

DIFFERENCE OF OPINION: YOUR DOCTOR MIGHT NOT BE RECEPTIVE

Clair's fertility specialist told her he thought she made the right decision. "He said, 'Oh, yeah, that's what I would do. Hours and hours of labor versus 15 minutes and you're done.' " Her obstetrician agreed. "He said, 'If that's what you want, that's what you should have. This is a team approach.' He didn't have a problem with it." A few weeks after Clair scheduled her cesarean, her daughter happened to turn into the breech position, providing a medical reason for the operation after all.

You might find that your doctor is less enthusiastic about the idea of your having an elective C-section. Doctors certainly have mixed views on the topic. When the American College of Obstetricians and Gynecologists, or ACOG, held a symposium on the subject in 2002, the planned 15-minute discussion period stretched into an hour. In a 2003 Gallup Organization survey of female OB/GYNs, more than a third said they would not perform an elective cesarean if their patient requested it. But just about a third of them said they *would* perform a patient-choice C-section if asked, while the remainder said their willingness would depend on the circumstances and the patient.

Some doctors think that performing cesareans on women who don't need them is tantamount to malpractice. Take Isabel's doctor. Pregnant with her first daughter, now 5, Isabel told her doctor at her first appointment that she wanted a C-section. Her reason might be a bit unusual—"I'm gay, and I can't even imagine a huge baby coming out down there"—but she was insistent. Isabel, now 42, told him from the beginning that she wanted a C-section. And he flat out told her: You can't do that. The question about whether Isabel could choose to have a cesarean delivery became moot when she discovered that her health insurance wouldn't cover it unless it was medically necessary.

For Isabel, the story has a happy ending, although many women would probably be less than thrilled to learn, as she did, that they needed a C-section after hours of labor because their baby was in distress. Worried that her baby was getting too big, Isabel's doctor induced labor a few days before her due date. She had an epidural and dilated to 8 centimeters when her doctor became concerned about the baby's safety. He could feel that the umbilical cord was wrapped around the baby's neck and head. Isabel was going to get her C-section after all. "I was thinking, 'Great. I'm so lucky!'" she recalls. "Everything always works out for me the way I need it to. You see, I get my C-section anyway. They should have just listened to me."

Since she'd already had one C-section, Isabel got no argument when she asked to schedule one for the delivery of her second daughter, now 2. "The first one was much harder than the second one, because with the first I didn't know what to expect," she says. And instead of giving birth around midnight, after hours of labor, Isabel delivered daughter number two the morning after a good night's sleep.

On the other end of the spectrum from Isabel's doctor are physicians who believe that C-sections are safer for babies and can protect moms against loss of bladder control, a prolapsed uterus, and other long-term problems associated with vaginal deliveries. "There should be two ways of delivering a baby: easy vaginal birth or easy cesarean birth," says D. Campbell Walters, M.D., a Mount Vernon, Illinois, OB/GYN and author of *Just Take It Out*, a self-published book that extols cesareans and hysterectomies. "The era of difficult vaginal birth should be behind us now. We now have an excellent alternative," says Walters.

In the middle are doctors who think women should have the right to choose how they deliver as long as they're fully informed of the risks and benefits of each option. That's where it gets tricky,

TALKING POINT

Not all doctors are open to the idea of performing a
C-section just because a patient wants one. If you're seriously considering this option, you need to raise the issue
with your doctor early on, because he's not obligated to
deliver you by cesarean just because you ask him to.
Hear what he has to say. You might change your mind,
or you might feel the need to get another opinion.

though. ACOG cautions that there is not yet extensive evidence
comparing the risks and benefits of purely elective cesareans with
vaginal deliveries. Unless you have a medical need for a C-section,
the organization's ethics committee opined in late 2003, your
doctor is under no obligation to perform one or even to bring up
the idea. "In almost all situations, the patient has a right to refuse
unwanted treatment," the ethics committee concluded. "She does
not, however, have a parallel right to demand treatment that the
physician believes is unwise or overly risky." The committee's
opinion infuriated organizations that advocate low-tech births, such
as Lamaze International and the American College of Nurse-
Midwives. Although ACOG didn't exactly come out with a ringing
endorsement of patient-choice cesareans, low-tech birth proponents
think the group still downplayed the risks to mothers and babies.

RISKIER BUSINESS FOR MOMS?
C-SECTIONS VERSUS VAGINAL DELIVERIES

Skeptics question whether all doctors—let alone their patients—
are fully informed about the documented risks of C-sections. "An

elective C-section is not like unzipping a zipper and zipping it back up again," says Carolyn Zelop, M.D., an OB/GYN at the University of Connecticut. "This is major abdominal surgery; but women are being led to believe that this is not a major procedure, and that it's completely safe for them and completely safe for their baby."

Thankfully, in the United States and other developed countries these days, complications from childbirth are rare, but research suggests that a number of them are more likely to occur as a result of a C-section than a vaginal delivery. For example:

- About 8 percent of women who have a cesarean develop an infection afterward, compared to about 2 percent of women who deliver vaginally.

- Only about 1 percent of women experience a serious hemorrhage after delivery, but this complication is four to eight times more common in women who had a C-section.

- About 7 or 8 out of every 10,000 women who had a C-section will need further surgery after delivery, while only 1 or 2 out of every 10,000 who gave birth vaginally will.

- About 4 percent of women who delivered by cesarean need intensive care afterward, compared to less than one-tenth of one percent of women who deliver vaginally.

- It's extremely rare for women to die as a result of childbirth, but some research suggests it's three to seven times more likely to happen with a C-section than with a vaginal delivery.

In emergencies, in which a baby or mother could die or be seriously hurt if a C-section is not performed immediately, the operation's benefits clearly outweigh its risks, whatever they may be. And in certain non-emergency situations, such as when the baby is breech, research has shown that a planned C-section can minimize the risk of complications. "As a high-risk obstetrician, I truly believe there's a place for the use of C-sections," says Zelop. But what if you have no apparent need for a cesarean? Some argue that's when the known risks of the surgery tip the scales in favor of your having a vaginal delivery. In 1998, the ethics committee of the International Federation of Gynecology and Obstetrics concluded that performing C-sections for non-medical reasons was not ethically justified. "There is no hard evidence on the relative risks and benefits of term cesarean delivery for non-medical reasons, as compared with vaginal delivery," the committee wrote.

Just 2 years later, though, Harer, then president of the American College of Obstetricians and Gynecologists, or ACOG, fueled the debate with an editorial in one of the organization's publications. "Perhaps the time has come when the risks, benefits, and costs are so balanced between cesarean and vaginal delivery that the deciding factor should simply be the mother's preference for how her baby is to be delivered," Harer wrote. He's still amazed at the reaction to his article, which he views as a strike for patient autonomy. "I was surprised with the virulence from people who found it offensive that women might make up their own minds about their risks," he says. "I got some real hate mail."

Ironically, Harer's editorial appeared the same month that an ACOG task force released a 59-page report, the product of 3 years' work, on how to lower the C-section rate. Harer's editorial "kind of took the wind out of our sails," says task force chair Roger Freeman, M.D., a professor of obstetrics and gynecology at the University of California, Irvine.

By 2003, the respected *New England Journal of Medicine* published

Looking Back

The earliest recorded case of a woman who survived a C-section was that of the brave Elisabeth Alespachin in 1500. Reportedly, the poor woman had labored for days at her home in Switzerland. A fleet of midwives and barbers—in those days, barbers practiced some medicine as well as cut hair—couldn't get that baby out the old-fashioned way.

But Elisabeth's baby wasn't delivered by some hotshot Renaissance surgeon. That baby was delivered by the dad, Jacob Nufer, professional pig castrator. Not only did Elisabeth survive the birth of their first child, but she reportedly went on to deliver four other single babies and one set of twins vaginally.

Skeptics suspect that Elisabeth and Jacob's firstborn actually grew outside her uterus, a rare occurrence that would make for an easier abdominal delivery. And some historians question whether the whole thing ever happened, because the tale wasn't written down until decades afterward.

a "sounding board" piece entitled "Elective Primary Cesarean Delivery." While your doctor shouldn't bring up the subject, there's nothing wrong with him agreeing to deliver your baby by C-section if you ask him to, wrote authors Howard Minkoff, M.D., and Frank Chervenak, M.D. Minkoff, on the OB/GYN faculty of the State University of New York Downstate Medical Center in Brooklyn, says the risks of a C-section are "remarkably less" than they were a generation ago. But, says Minkoff, while "an informed patient should have the right to have her voice heard, I would attempt to dissuade someone from doing it."

If any mom-to-be could truly be fully informed about C-sections, you'd think it would be an obstetrician. In that recent Gallup poll of American female OB/GYNs, more than one in five of those who had had their own babies by cesarean said there had been no medical reason for it. "My best friend is an OB/GYN. She told me she thinks labor is barbaric," says Michele Lauria, M.D., an OB/GYN at Dartmouth Medical School. Her friend has never had children, Lauria says, but if she did, "she told me she would present in labor and tell them she was having a herpes outbreak," which some research suggests is reason enough for performing a C-section.

In recent months, says Miami OB/GYN Javier Vizoso, M.D., he's performed C-sections on two doctor colleagues and the wife of a third—who happens to be a labor-and-delivery nurse—all at the patients' request. One of the two medical centers at which Vizoso directs obstetrics and gynecology, South Miami Hospital, had the highest cesarean rate in Florida: 42 percent in 2001. But if he were a woman and pregnant for the first time, Vizoso says, he would at least try to deliver vaginally. When patients ask for a cesarean, he ticks off some of the risks associated with abdominal surgery:

* Internal bleeding that may require a blood transfusion
* Injuries to the bowel, bladder, and other internal organs (not to mention the uterus)
* Blood clots
* Infection

"I don't let people off the hook easily," he says. Still, Vizoso acknowledges, "no matter how much I try to discourage them, my rate of convincing them to try a vaginal delivery is pretty low." Even if you've pretty much made up your mind that you want to have a C-section, at least keep an open mind when you discuss the matter with your doctor.

Words from the Wise

Although C-sections are safer than ever, they carry the same risks as other major abdominal operations, such as blood clots and infection. That's more than a fair tradeoff if medical reasons necessitate a speedy delivery. But if your baby, like most, could safely be delivered vaginally, some doctors question whether the risks of a cesarean are worth it.

PLANNING AHEAD:
PREPLANNED VERSUS UNPLANNED C-SECTIONS

You might be thinking of going ahead and scheduling a cesarean because you figure it's got to be safer than undergoing one at the last minute after hours of labor. That sounds logical, but few studies distinguish between the two. As a result, what appear to be complications of cesareans may actually be related to protracted labor or the factors leading to it. Such complications might have been prevented if the C-section had been planned instead of an emergency. "We've saved their lives by doing a C-section," Walters says. "When they have a complication, we blame the C-section."

One advantage of planning your C-section is that it's likely to take place during bankers' hours. When you deliver vaginally, especially if your labor isn't induced, you don't have much say about when your baby is born. Some older studies, done in the 1970s, suggested that the timing of a delivery could affect its outcome. Babies born during the daytime and on weekdays, when doctors, nurses, and other hospital staff tend to be more rested and numerous, were found to have lower death rates than babies born at night or on weekends. More recent research findings about the time of day or day of the week have been inconsistent, though. In a study of nearly 700,000 births, published in 2003, scientists from Stockholm's Karolinska Institute found that babies born at night had a higher risk of dying shortly after birth than babies born during the day. (Remember, though, few babies died overall, so the difference in the actual number of deaths between the two groups was quite small.) However, another huge study—this one of more than 1.6 million live births in California—found no evidence that the quality of care before, during, or after delivery was compromised on weekends.

For the most part, pre-planned C-sections appear to be safer and, not surprisingly, more acceptable to moms than unplanned emergency C-sections. Recent research by obstetricians at the University of Vienna in Austria suggests that as far as psychological factors, pain levels, and birth experience, there's no comparison between the two types of C-sections.

Words from the Wise

Generally, planned C-sections are safer than unplanned C-sections.

Using questionnaires and psychological tests, the researchers evaluated 1,050 pregnant women 2 weeks before their due date and 3 days and again at 4 months after delivery. A total of 147 women delivered by planned cesarean—3 for medical reasons and 44 at the patients' request. Another 93 women had unplanned C-sections. The women who had elective cesareans reported having the best birth experience, while the 41 who had vaginal deliveries with vacuum extraction reported having the worst. The researchers concluded that elective C-sections were safe and "psychologically well-tolerated," and that the results were similar to uncomplicated vaginal deliveries.

In a recent study of more than 18,000 pregnancies, Nova Scotia researchers found that if you deliver by a planned C-section, you tend to fare better overall than if you deliver by emergency C-section or vaginally with the help of forceps or vacuum extraction. The scientists identified only one minor drawback to preplanned cesareans: Afterward, you're twice as likely to run a fever of more than 100.4 degrees than if you had labored before delivering. Still, your actual risk of an elevated temperature is pretty low. Fewer than 1 percent of all women in the study developed a fever.

This is reassuring: A University of Washington study suggests that planned C-sections are just as safe as vaginal deliveries, at least as far as your risk of dying afterward, which is extremely low to begin with. Only 11 out of the 265,471 women in this study died of pregnancy-related causes within 6 months of giving birth. After accounting for advanced maternal age and severe preeclampsia, there was no difference in pregnancy-related death rates between the C-section group and the vaginal delivery group. The researchers concluded that it wasn't C-sections that raised the risk of dying, but the medical conditions that necessitated them.

In a separate report, though, the researchers did find one disadvantage to having a cesarean: If you deliver by that route, you may be nearly twice as likely to require re-hospitalization within the next 2 months as women who deliver vaginally without the help of forceps or vacuum extraction. Once again, the overall risk appears to be exceedingly low. Just over 1 percent of the more than 250,000 women in the study had to go back into the hospital within 2 months of delivering their babies. Common reasons for re-hospitalization were uterine infections, wound complications, and blood clots.

Chances are excellent that you won't need to be re-hospitalized after having a C-section, but you probably won't return to your normal activities as quickly as you would after a vaginal delivery. The University of Washington researchers found that about two-thirds of first-time moms who had a spontaneous—no forceps or vacuum extraction—vaginal delivery said they could perform vigorous activities such as running, lifting heavy objects, and participating in strenuous sports by 7 weeks after giving birth. Just under half of the women who delivered by C-section felt the same way. Interestingly, normal household tasks seemed to be more of a challenge than pumping iron or sweating it out on the track or tennis court: Only half of the women who had unassisted vaginal deliveries and a third of those who had C-sections said they could do routine chores around the house without difficulty.

Hmmm. Either this finding illustrates the psychological component of recovery, or the women's homes must have really been a mess. After the cesarean delivery of her first daughter,

> **Words from the Wise**
>
> *Recovery tends to take longer after a C-section than after a vaginal delivery.*

now age 3, 26-year-old Jaime says, "I was in so much pain, I couldn't do anything when I went home. I could hardly lift my daughter." Jaime's C-section came after 3 days of labor, which may have slowed her recovery. Clair, on the other hand, was an exception to those University of Washington research findings. For her, ecstasy over finally becoming a mother worked better than any painkiller ever could after her elective C-section. "I knew it would be harder for me to recover, but I bounced back pretty quickly," she says. "I was literally fine 3 to 4 weeks afterward. I felt great."

Some doctors are concerned that higher numbers of patient-choice cesareans could reveal long-term problems with the procedure that haven't yet surfaced. A small Brazilian study might provide an inkling of what's to come in the United States. Brazil's C-section delivery rate is the highest in the world, and the majority are scheduled without a pressing medical reason. Among women in the higher socioeconomic groups, at least, C-sections greatly outnumber vaginal deliveries. You might relate to at least some of the reasons for C-sections' popularity in Brazil, although you might not call them unjustified, as a Sao Paulo OB/GYN did in a letter a few years ago to *BMJ,* a British medical journal.

"Some unjustified fears cause this situation, including the fear of fetal distress during labor, the notion that labor lasting more than 6 hours is unbearable for the mother, the fear that a vaginal delivery will ruin the woman's sex life, and the idea that a cesarean section is better and more 'modern,' since it is the preferred form of delivery for rich women in our country. The patients also want to plan the day of the birth, choosing a relative's birthday or avoiding a holiday, for instance."

Colleagues of the letter-writer at the University of Sao Paulo blame the over-use of cesareans to a rise in cases of chronic pelvic pain seen at their hospital. They reached that conclusion after comparing 116 patients who underwent a laparoscopy for the diagnosis of chronic pelvic pain with 83 patients who didn't have pain, but who underwent a laparoscopy to have their tubes tied. Two-thirds of the women with chronic pelvic pain had had a C-section, compared to a little more than a third of the women without pain. "I am convinced that cesarean section can be a cause of chronic pelvic pain," says co-author Antonio Alberto Nogueira, M.D. At his hospital, Nogueira says, he's seen an increase in patients with chronic pelvic pain who've had two or more C-sections. You might think this would never happen to you if you had a C-section, and you probably would be right. But it might be one more thing to consider when weighing the pros and cons of requesting a C-section.

GOTTA GO:
DO VAGINAL BIRTHS DELIVER
A LIFETIME OF PELVIC FLOOR WOES?

If you're like many women choosing cesareans, the explanation is as simple as this: You don't ever want to wear the diapers in the family. Maybe you've already experienced incontinence during your pregnancy—leaking urine every time you laugh or cough, or feeling like you need to run to the bathroom more frequently than a newly potty-trained toddler. How could a vaginal delivery not make things worse?

The subject is so anxiety-provoking that it made perfect fodder for an episode of *Frasier*. Julia, the radio psychiatrist's tactless girlfriend *du jour*, spills the beans that Niles and Daphne are expecting. "Two words: C-section," Julia advises Daphne. "My sister's about your size, and when she had her kids, it blew out the whole region."

Intuitively, it does make sense that pushing a baby through your vagina must wreak havoc on your pelvic floor, the hammock of muscles that supports the pelvic organs. According to one study, women with a normal life expectancy have an 11 percent chance of undergoing surgery for pelvic organ prolapse—in which the uterus, bladder, rectum, or small intestine protrude into the vagina, causing discomfort and incontinence—or urinary incontinence at some point in their lives.

No question, if you deliver vaginally, you're more likely to have a bladder control problem afterward than if you have a C-section. That might be enough to make you want to schedule a cesarean, but it's not

Looking Back

There's a difference of opinion about who gets credit for performing the first successful C-section in the United States. One camp says it was Dr. Jesse Bennett of Virginia, who reportedly delivered his own child by cesarean in 1794 and then promptly removed his wife's ovaries so he (and she, we suppose) would never have to go through that again. But others credit John Lambert Richmond, physician and Baptist minister. The date: April 22, 1827, exactly 5 years after Richmond graduated from medical school. The location: a backwoods cabin in, of course, Ohio. The woman had been in labor for 30 hours, but her cervix hadn't dilated at all. Richmond used "common pocket instruments" to deliver her baby via cesarean. "She commenced work in 24 days from the operation, and in the fifth week walked a mile and back the same day," he reported afterward.

as bad as it sounds. In a study of 595 pregnant women, researchers from Dalhousie University in Halifax, Nova Scotia, looked at rates of incontinence up to 6 months after delivery. Six months after giving birth, 10 percent of those who had undergone C-sections reported having urinary incontinence, compared to 22 percent of those who had spontaneous vaginal deliveries and 33 percent of those who delivered vaginally with the help of forceps. Though urinary incontinence was twice as common in women who had spontaneous vaginal deliveries than in women who had C-sections, most of those affected said they could live with it. Overall, only about 3.5 percent of incontinent women—three women out of the entire study of 595—said it was limiting their activities.

You can get some idea about your chances of becoming incontinent after the birth by looking at whether you're wetting your pants or frequently running to the bathroom while pregnant. All other things being equal, you're twice as likely to be incontinent after delivery if you're incontinent while pregnant, according to a recently published study of 523 women by researchers in Birmingham, Alabama, and Pittsburgh. Mode of delivery has a similar effect on your risk of incontinence, at least through baby's first birthday, the study found. If you deliver vaginally, it suggests, you're twice as likely to be incontinent than if you have a cesarean. The difference persisted for at least a year after birth, but you have to remember that only about 10 percent of all the study participants were still incontinent at that time. Although the proportion of women who were incontinent remained pretty stable during the year after delivery, they had fewer and fewer accidents over time. The study also provides another reason (as if you needed one!) to stop smoking and get down to a reasonable weight before you conceive: Both smoking and being overweight raised the risk of incontinence after delivery. Some research suggests that smoking increases the likelihood of incontinence by causing chronic coughing, and scientists speculate that excess weight places extra pressure on the pelvic floor.

Incontinence might not develop until years after delivery, so researchers have found it a challenge to study an association between the two. Because incontinence is rare before age 50, much of the research that currently exists focuses on women who gave birth years ago, when the management of labor and delivery was quite different than it is today, notes Catherine Spong, M.D., director of perinatology research at the National Institute for Child Health and Human Development, part of the National Institutes of Health. "I don't think you can compare what happened then and what's happening now in incontinence issues," Spong says.

Still, many urogynecologists—doctors who specialize in treating women for incontinence—are convinced that cesareans protect against pelvic floor problems. That's why urologist Jennifer Berman opted for a C-section for the delivery of her second child. Berman delivered daughter Isabelle live on a Discovery Health Channel special. On *Good Morning America* and the Discovery channel's Web site, Berman explained that she chose to have a cesarean because her first delivery had been so difficult. Son Max, who weighed in at a whopping 9½ pounds, was born after 18 hours of labor and hours of pushing. As a result, Berman said, she experienced incontinence for 7 months

Words from the Wise

If you're having bladder control issues while pregnant, research suggests that you're more likely to have them after you deliver, whether by C-section or vaginally. But even if you do experience incontinence after delivery, it tends to become less of a problem over time.

after his birth and during her second pregnancy. "I was just really adamant that I didn't want to go through that again, or suffer the consequences down below, so to speak."

Unfortunately for Berman, the horse was probably already out of the barn by the time she scheduled a C-section for Isabelle's delivery. Research suggests that women are most likely to sustain pelvic floor damage as a result of their first vaginal delivery, not subsequent ones.

Kim, a Denver OB/GYN, knew years before she was ever pregnant that she wanted to deliver by cesarean. She'd operated on enough women whose uterus eventually sagged into their vagina after delivering a baby through that opening. "I saw the effects of vaginal delivery and was definitely tainted," says Kim, who recently had her first child at age 35.

If you have similar concerns, keep in mind that C-sections don't prevent pelvic floor problems altogether. Simply carrying a baby those last few months of pregnancy, no matter how it's delivered, seems to increase the risk of incontinence. So does just getting older.

A recent study of more than 15,000 Norwegian women under age 65 found that those who had never had a baby had the lowest risk of urinary incontinence. Compared to them, women who had only had cesareans were about 50 percent more likely to be incontinent. And those who had only had vaginal deliveries were twice as likely to be incontinent as those who had never had a baby. "I think important new knowledge from our study

Words from the Wise

If you've already had a vaginal delivery, opting to deliver by C-section the next time around may not have much effect on your risk of incontinence.

is that pregnancy in itself is a risk factor for incontinence," says lead author Guri Rortveit, M.D., a general practice doctor at the University of Bergen.

But you have to remember that incontinence is not terribly common, especially in women under 50.

> **Words from the Wise**
>
> *Simply being pregnant raises your risk of incontinence, no matter how you deliver. So does getting older. Still, the majority of women who deliver vaginally don't experience incontinence.*

And by age 50, incontinence was just about as common in the cesarean group as in the vaginal delivery group, Rortveit's team found. According to the Norwegian researchers, if you delivered all of your children by cesarean, your risk of moderate to severe urinary incontinence would drop from 10 percent to 5 percent. That's not a good enough reason to opt for a cesarean, Rortveit says, because you're unlikely to develop incontinence even if you deliver vaginally. To prevent incontinence in one woman, Rortveit says, 13 women would have to deliver all of their children by C-section.

The sad but true fact is that even women who have never given birth can become incontinent as they age. University of Rochester researchers demonstrated that with a study of 149 nuns, average age 68. None of the nuns had ever given birth. The scientists surveyed the nuns about whether they currently had a problem with urine loss and, if so, how much it impacted their life. Nearly half of the nuns reported having a problem with urinary incontinence, and nearly all said they were bothered by it. For more than two-thirds of them, the problem had been going on for years. Half of the incontinent nuns said they needed to wear sanitary pads to protect their clothing. So much for thinking that the greatest risk factor for incontinence is damage from a vaginal delivery!

Bottom line, research into the impact of mode of delivery on incontinence risk suggests that delivering via C-section instead of vaginally might, at most, delay incontinence for a small percentage of women. Which would not be such a bad thing, says Roger Goldberg, M.D., director of urogynecology research at the Evanston Continence Center in Evanston, Illinois. As Rochester researchers found, many women are incontinent by age 60, so their childbearing history, or lack thereof, might not have much effect by that point, Goldberg says. Instead, he says, "I think perhaps we are dealing with quality of life between 30 and 60."

It's difficult to predict which women will develop pelvic floor problems as a result of giving birth vaginally. But some doctors suggest that you ask your mother about her experience. If she experienced prolapse or stress incontinence—the leaking of urine when she laughed or coughed—after delivering you vaginally, you might be more likely to as well. But remember, the majority of women who deliver vaginally, including those who have many children, do not experience incontinence.

Rochester urogynecologist Gunhilde Buchsbaum, M.D., suspects that incontinence runs in families; but, as her nun study suggests, it may not matter how you deliver or if you ever gave birth at all. For more evidence, she cites her ongoing study of pairs of postmenopausal sisters. In each pair, one sister had given birth, the other never had. Buchsbaum has found no association between having a baby and risk of incontinence. But she did find that in two-thirds of the sister pairs, either both were incontinent or neither was. Of the pairs in which only one was incontinent, half the time it was the sister who had never given birth. Happily, Buchsbaum points out, incontinence now can often be treated with techniques that are far less invasive than a C-section.

FEAR AND LABORING: ANXIETY MAY PLAY A ROLE IN DEMAND FOR C-SECTIONS

If you think a C-section seems like the easier route to motherhood, you're not alone. About 6 to 10 percent of pregnant women have a severe fear of childbirth, often leading them to request a cesarean. They represent about 7 to 22 percent (depending on what study you read) of C-sections performed in Finland, Sweden, and the United Kingdom, Finnish researchers found. And the situation is probably not that different in the United States. "I do see people in class absolutely panicked," says Marguerite Truesdale, a childbirth educator at Beth Israel Hospital in Boston. "Intellectually, they know they're pregnant, but they haven't really thought a lot about how this baby is going to come out." Stunned, they tell Truesdale: "The baby's coming out where?! Sign me up for a cesarean!"

Like Berman, Alexes chose to deliver her second child by C-section. She was concerned about loss of bladder control after a lengthy labor with her first baby. But you can't help but wonder whether that was the only reason why she wanted to schedule a cesarean delivery. "My feeling is it should be an option," Alexes, a plastic surgeon, told a Pittsburgh newspaper several months after her C-section. "My attitude about childbirth is that there's this whole crazy movement—and there has been for awhile—toward natural childbirth . . . getting no anesthesia, getting no medicine, because somehow medicine is bad. So women are forced to go through this barbaric ritual, and I think it's insane."

Resistance to anesthesia in childbirth dates back to when general anesthesia with nitrous oxide or ether was first demonstrated in the mid-19th century. There were those who actually thought it was immoral to eliminate pain, especially in childbirth. It practically took a royal decree to dispel that notion. In 1853, an English physician administered chloroform to Queen Victoria before delivering her eighth child.

More than 150 years later, epidural anesthesia provides excellent relief if the pain of labor, which can go on for hours, becomes unbearable. And, unlike Queen Victoria, you get to remain awake for your baby's birth. Spong, of the National Institutes of Health, can't understand why some women still think they have to suffer to deliver a baby vaginally. "I've gotten some e-mails from people saying that childbirth was the most excruciating thing that they'd ever gone through," she says. "They'd tell all their friends not to have children. I find it very sad when people say that." Dartmouth's Michele Lauria, M.D., points out, "I've never seen anybody lose it from the pain of labor. Nobody ever kind of jumps out of their skin and dies from the pain."

Dawn, 34, was just never a fan of having too many people "down there." Before she got pregnant, she had to grit her teeth to make it through routine pelvic exams. The only way she could ever imagine delivering a baby was by C-section. She'd heard it might be safer for the baby, but fear of a vaginal delivery was the driving force behind her desire to have a cesarean. "For me, it was the only

TALKING POINT

If you're so anxious about labor that you're thinking of scheduling a C-section simply to avoid it, talk to your doctor about the excellent options available for pain relief.

option. I've always been kind of a chicken." When she did become pregnant, Dawn made sure to pick an obstetrician who had a reputation for scheduling cesareans if patients wanted them. Dawn says, "I didn't give her an option." And the doctor never tried to talk her out of it; she understood how Dawn felt. So did her husband. Since Dawn was carrying the baby, he felt she should decide how it was going to come out.

For the most part, though, Dawn was kind of embarrassed to share her feelings with others while she was pregnant. "I didn't really let it be known publicly what I was going to do. People do almost look at you badly," she says. "Now I'll tell people straight out: It was either that or no baby." She found it a strange coincidence that all 10 women in the "Mommy and Me" class she attended after her daughter's birth had delivered by C-section. Dawn didn't for a minute believe that she was the only one who chose to have a cesarean. "I just think I'm more honest than most people. I've never had anyone openly admit it to me, but I know for a fact there are women who have had it voluntarily."

Dawn skipped attending a childbirth education course, figuring it would be a waste for her. And the hospital where she planned to deliver didn't offer a C-section class. Still, "I wanted to be somewhat educated about what was going to happen to me. I've never had major surgery before. I didn't know exactly what it involved." Toward that end, she read books and watched what she calls "the greatest television." Despite her fear of a vaginal delivery, Dawn became addicted to the labor-and-delivery shows on cable TV, which show both C-sections and vaginal births. She also asked friends who'd had cesareans to describe their experiences in detail.

Yet, it was nothing like she expected. "Okay. I read a lot of books. They say this is what a C-section is, and this is what happens. They don't make light of it, but they don't tell you how serious it is. It was more of a surgery than I expected." The most disappointing part:

Words from the Wise

You might be tempted to bone up on labor and delivery by watching the increasingly popular TV shows on the subject. But this is one type of reality programming you might want to skip (try Survivor *or* American Idol *instead), at least until after your own delivery, and this is why: Some of the shows can be pretty graphic and scary to some people. If you're somewhat anxious about labor and delivery, at least ask a friend to tape a show and screen it before you watch.*

"Right after I had her, I never really got to see her. I just didn't get to look at her long enough. After all this time, I just wanted to see her. They took her away. They cleaned her up and all. I didn't see her until maybe 3 or 4 hours later. I was asking about her."

Dawn most likely could have delivered vaginally. Her daughter, now 13 months, wasn't breech and weighed just under 6 pounds. If she ever has another child—and that's a big if—she'll attempt a vaginal delivery.

OH, BABY: THE RISKS AND BENEFITS OF C-SECTIONS FOR NEWBORNS

Pain isn't the only anxiety-provoking aspect of labor and delivery. Many women who ask for a C-section are haunted by stories of babies left profoundly handicapped because of a vaginal delivery gone awry. Or they've heard about the extremely rare case of a woman who died in childbirth. As recently as 1968, though, the C-section rate in the United States was only around 5 percent, notes Kaiser Permanente OB/GYN Bruce Flamm, M.D., of Riverside, California. "Were a lot of women dying in labor?" he asks. "No."

But what about the babies? "I had a friend in college whose brother was severely handicapped as a result of a traumatic birth," says Jean, 42, who asked for a cesarean at one of her first prenatal visits. "In that situation, the parents had resisted the obstetrician's advice to perform a C-section. By the time of my second pregnancy, I also had a friend who had lost a baby at birth because a C-section was not done in a timely manner."

With Jean's first pregnancy 11 years ago, her doctor told her she couldn't have a cesarean without a good medical reason. "But in due course, there was: my daughter was in a footling breech position," Jean says. "My doctor said, 'Well, it looks like you're going to get that cesarean.'" When she became pregnant with her son 7 years later, Jean says, she again asked her doctor for a C-section, even though she was a good candidate for a vaginal birth. "It's fine with me," said the doctor, who, since delivering Jean's firstborn by cesarean, had her own baby by C-section.

"I'm not saying that every woman should demand a scheduled C-section," Jean says. "I'm saying that 'natural birth' advocates should stop wailing about mothers' empowerment long enough to consider the children. We don't procreate so that we can experience birth; we procreate to have children to love and raise."

Still, current research suggests that, for single babies who are full-term and head-down, vaginal deliveries generally are at least as safe as planned C-sections. There's no difference in the risk of death, and there's no evidence that a cesarean reduces the already extremely low risk—about 2 per 10,000—of neurological problems such as cerebral palsy caused by a problem during labor.

BREATHING LESSONS:
LABOR HELPS PRIME BABIES' LUNGS

Clearly, babies delivered by C-section have a higher risk of a respiratory condition called transient tachypnea of the neonate, or TTN for short. TTN is also called "wet lungs" or type II respiratory distress syndrome. It occurs in about 1 percent of all newborns, but in 4 percent of those delivered by cesarean. The symptoms of TTN, such as rapid, labored breathing and a grunting sound when the baby exhales, appear within a few hours of birth. As its name suggests, TTN usually lasts only a few days, but it's probably one of the main reasons babies are admitted to intensive care nurseries. "In the long run, nothing terrible happens, but you're supposed to be bonding with your baby, and they're taking your baby to the NICU (neonatal intensive care unit)," says OB/GYN Cynthia Holcroft, M.D., of Johns Hopkins University in Baltimore.

TTN, which is treated with oxygen therapy, results from too much fluid in the baby's lungs. It's thought that the pressure of passing through the birth canal helps squeeze out the fluid, which may at least partially explain why TTN is more common in babies delivered by C-section. In addition, labor itself sets off a stress response in newborns, triggering the production of the hormone epinephrine, which also helps clear out fluid. That may be why TTN is even more common in babies delivered by planned C-sections performed before labor begins.

Another contributing factor to TTN might be the timing of elective cesareans. Scheduling C-sections is tricky. If you're definitely going to deliver by cesarean, you probably want to avoid going into labor. In a post on CaesareanBirth.com, Sue writes about going into labor 3 days before her planned C-section. "I was having very hard contractions," she writes. "By the time the doctor arrived, I was dilated to 10 centimeters and just minutes from a breech birth. I am pregnant again and have already informed my doctor that I do not, under any circumstances, wish to go into labor. He agrees, and hopefully we are going to schedule this one sooner than the last."

Doctors tend to schedule cesareans around the 38th or 39th week of pregnancy. They don't want to deliver the baby prematurely, which doesn't happen as often as it used to, thanks to improved methods of assessing gestational age. To make sure your due date is correct, your doctor will look at when you had a positive pregnancy test and the results of your ultrasounds. Even in full-term pregnancies, just 1 or 2 weeks can make a difference in the baby's health, according to a study by obstetricians at the University College London Medical School. Among newborns delivered before labor began, those born at 37 to 37½ weeks were 2½ times more likely to develop TTN or respiratory distress syndrome than those delivered at 39 or 39½ weeks. Babies are considered to be full-term anywhere from 37 to 40 weeks gestation.

While TTN appears to have no long-lasting effect, research may not yet be complete. There are very few data, to my knowledge, that actually follow up large numbers of children with TTN," says Gordon Smith, M.D., Ph.D., of Cambridge University in Britain. He presented the results of one such study at the annual meeting of the Society for Gynecological Investigation. Smith and his collaborators looked at nearly 175,000 full-term births at Scottish hospitals. Compared to children delivered vaginally, those delivered by planned cesarean who developed TTN were more likely to be hospitalized for asthma or a respiratory tract infection when they were 5 to 9 years old. A separate study of 31-year-old adults in Finland found that those delivered by

TALKING POINT

If you're planning to deliver by C-section, schedule it as late in your pregnancy as possible to minimize your baby's chance of having breathing problems.

C-section (researchers lumped planned and unplanned together) were more than three times more likely to have asthma than those delivered vaginally.

A team of Chicago researchers reviewed nearly 30,000 consecutive deliveries over a period of 7 years at their hospital to examine the risk of respiratory problems in newborns. They found that babies delivered by preplanned cesarean were almost five times more likely to be diagnosed with a rare condition called persistent pulmonary hypertension, in which blood vessels in the lungs fail to dilate and allow the proper flow of oxygen to other organs. The actual rate of primary pulmonary hypertension was just under 4 per 1,000 live births among the planned C-section babies, compared to 0.8 per 1,000 live births among babies delivered vaginally. After being placed on a respirator and given oxygen, most, but not all, affected babies do okay. "Mortality is very low, but it's not zero," says lead author Elliot Levine. "That's the problem. Fortunately, we don't see it that often, but the fact that we see it more often in sectioned patients than in vaginally delivered patients means cesarean is not that benign." Yet, he says, that consent form you sign for a C-section overlooks such risks to the baby.

As far as some types of delivery-related injuries are concerned, cesareans performed before labor begins appear to be as safe for babies as vaginal deliveries. Take cuts. Remember, C-sections involve incisions, and sometimes the baby as well as the mother gets cut. Researchers at the Naval Medical Center in San Diego reviewed all charts of babies delivered at their hospital over a 4-year period who sustained a cut during cesarean delivery. Babies were cut in about one

Words from the Wise

Labor can be beneficial to your baby's lungs.

out of every 133 C-sections, but the injuries were associated with a laboring uterus.

A study of nearly 600,000 first babies born to California women examined the effect of mode of delivery on the risk of brain injuries, which, you should know, are rare complications. Of the women who had C-sections, more than a quarter delivered before they went into labor. Brain hemorrhages occurred in 1 of every 2,750 babies delivered by cesarean with no labor, about the same rate as in babies delivered vaginally without the help of forceps or vacuum extraction.

If you have food allergies, here's one more thing to think about when debating whether to ask for a C-section: A recent study published by scientists with the Norwegian Institute of Public Health suggests that children delivered by C-section have a greater risk of developing food allergies than those delivered vaginally. Researchers asked the parents of 2,803 children whether they appeared to be allergic to eggs, fish or nuts at age 2½. The scientists also tested children reported to be allergic to eggs. They found no connection between mode of delivery and risk of food allergies in kids whose mothers weren't allergic. But allergic mothers who delivered by cesarean were seven times more likely to report that their toddlers had food allergies than allergic mothers who delivered vaginally. Apparently, it wasn't all in the allergic mothers' heads, either. The kids delivered by C-section were also four times more likely to have a doctor-confirmed egg allergy than those delivered vaginally. Again, there was no such association among children of women who weren't allergic. So how could delivery by C-section increase your baby's risk of inheriting your food allergies? The researchers speculate that cesarean delivery might delay healthful bacteria (yes, there are such microbes) from taking up residence in newborns' guts. Such a delay might play a role in the development of food allergies. Something to consider if eating eggs makes you break out in hives.

DOWN THE ROAD: C-SECTIONS COULD AFFECT FUTURE PREGNANCIES

You could skip the next section if you're planning on having only one child. But if you're thinking about having more than one, you should know that choosing to have a cesarean might impact future pregnancies or your likelihood of even conceiving. If you're thinking about having four or more children, you should think twice about scheduling a C-section simply because you want one.

With each cesarean, your risk of placenta complications increases. Some, but not all, research suggests that your risk of experiencing a tear in your uterus increases with each cesarean. And some research suggests that you might have a harder time getting pregnant after a C-section than after a vaginal delivery.

Placenta previa, in which the placenta covers all or part of the cervix, occurs in about one in 200 births, or half a percent. After one cesarean, though, your risk of placenta previa in your next pregnancy is 1 percent to 4 percent. Having placenta previa and one prior C-section increases your risk of a potentially life-threatening problem called placenta accreta to 25 percent in your next pregnancy. In placenta accreta, the placenta burrows itself into the uterine wall, so it usually must be surgically removed after delivery. Placenta accreta can cause vaginal bleeding in the third trimester, although in most cases there are no symptoms until delivery, which is often premature. According to the American College of Obstetricians and Gynecologists, placenta accreta is now 10 times more common than it was 50 years ago, most likely because of the increasing cesarean delivery rate. This OB/GYN group says placenta accreta occurs in one out of every 2,500 deliveries, but some doctors believe it is more common that that. Two thirds of women with placenta accreta will need to have an emergency hysterectomy to stem the bleeding that can occur when the doctor tries to separate the placenta from the uterus. Up to 7 percent of women with placenta accreta die.

Placenta abnormalities, such as placenta accreta, are the main reason women need an emergency hysterectomy right after delivery. Such procedures are rare, occurring in one to three out of every 1,000 deliveries in the United States. But they're even less common in countries that have lower cesarean delivery rates. Placenta abnormalities also might increase the risk of stillbirth in pregnant women who previously delivered by cesarean, Smith theorizes. In a study of nearly 121,000 Scottish births, Smith found that women who had a prior C-section were about 64 percent more likely to have an unexplained stillbirth in their next pregnancy than women who'd had a previous vaginal delivery. That translated into rates of 2.4 stillbirths per 10,000 women per week versus 1.5 per 10,000 women per week. The increased risk of stillbirth began at around 34 weeks into the pregnancy after a cesarean, and it was the same no matter why that C-section was performed. The association between prior cesarean and stillbirth was even stronger when limited to women whose first baby was born at or after 40 weeks gestation. Still, Smith and his collaborators emphasize that, on average, your chance of delivering a stillborn baby after a prior C-section is only around one in 1,100, compared to 1 in 2,000 for women who previously had delivered vaginally. And if there's a medical reason for a C-section—say, if your baby is breech—the benefits outweigh the higher risk of stillbirth in a subsequent pregnancy.

As the worldwide cesarean delivery rate has risen over the past 2 decades, so has the number of couples seeking help for infertility, leading researchers to wonder whether there is a connection between the two.

Research by Maureen Porter, M.D., an OB/GYN at the University of Aberdeen in Scotland, suggests that women who have trouble getting pregnant after a C-section probably had trouble getting pregnant before it—so it's not like the operation damaged their reproductive organs in any way. But, Porter says, the main reason women don't get pregnant after having a cesarean is because they don't want to. "Our findings suggest that it is often connected to the experience of cesarean section or the events around it," she says. Porter, who has reported her results at international infertility conferences, acknowledges that the findings don't necessarily apply to women who chose to deliver by C-section, as opposed to those who delivered by emergency cesareans after a prolonged labor. Many of the 1,117 women in Porter's study said they decided to put off having more children after a prior C-section because they felt that labor had gone on too long before the operation was finally performed. But, even an elective C-section carries psychological risks, Porter notes. In her research, some women said they delayed getting pregnant again because recovery from their cesarean was much longer or more difficult than expected, an experience all women who undergo C-sections—whether preplanned or emergency—might relate to. If you wait too long to conceive after a cesarean, Porter notes, your

Words from the Wise

Of course, when you're pregnant, your top concern is the baby you are carrying, not any future children you might have. But if you're considering scheduling a C-section for the sake of convenience, not your health or your baby's, you should know that there's a chance it could adversely impact future pregnancies.

voluntary infertility might become involuntary because of your age. On the face of it, choosing a C-section might seem tempting. But, as you can see from this chapter, it is not a decision to be made lightly. If you have no compelling medical reason to schedule a cesarean, some experts would argue, the operation's risks outweigh its benefits. Others would point out that C-sections are safer than ever, so you should be allowed to go that route even if you don't really have to. Clearly, no one else can decide what's best for you. But you need to be as fully informed as possible—talk to your doctor, talk to other women about their experiences, talk to a childbirth educator—before making the important choice about how to deliver your baby.

CHAPTER 5

BE PREPARED

When you want to avoid a C-Section

Barbara's long-time obstetrician knew she wanted neither a C-section nor an epidural for her second son, born 8 years after her first, when she was 44. "I've had enough surgeries," says Barbara, now 47, who dealt with years of infertility treatments. "I thought if you're so uncomfortable from your own surgery, how can you truly be bonding with your baby? I just didn't want the clinical delivery."

Pulling off an unmedicated vaginal delivery wasn't easy. The baby was sideways, but Barbara's doctor managed to turn him head-down— the best position for a vaginal delivery— and hold him there for 45 minutes to make sure he didn't roll back on his side. She then sat patiently with Barbara through hours of labor. When the baby's heart rate slowed precipitously, Barbara's doctor didn't rush to perform an emergency cesarean. When the time was right, and at her doctor's command, Barbara quickly pushed her son out.

If you're African-American, at least 40 years old, or less than 5-foot-1, research suggests that you have a higher chance of delivering by C-section than a woman who's Caucasian, under age 40 or 5-foot-1 or taller—all other things being equal. Now, of course, you have no control over your race, your age, or your height. But if you've weighed the pros and cons and decided you'd prefer to deliver vaginally—and you have no pressing medical reasons not to—there are steps you can take to minimize your chances of having an unplanned C-section. "Educating yourself is important and can play a key role in preventing a cesarean," Jaime, who has had two, writes on CaesareanBirth.com, the Web site she launched after her second. "It might be the last thing you want to think about; but thinking ahead can be what keeps you off the operating table."

Remember, most cesareans are unplanned, so no one can guarantee that you'll get your wish for a vaginal delivery. Should something unforeseen occur and you end up delivering by cesarean, you can take comfort knowing that you did what was in your power to avoid it. And, as this book will regularly remind you, there is no reason to feel like you've failed if your delivery doesn't go the way you'd hoped it would.

A GOOD FIT: FIND A HOSPITAL AND DOCTOR WHO SHARE YOUR PHILOSOPHY

This may seem pretty obvious, but it bears repeating: If you want to avoid a C-section, look for a hospital and a doctor with low C-section rates, preferably 15 percent or less for first-time moms delivering full-term, head-down babies. (Remember that hospitals and doctors with a preponderance of high-risk patients may have higher C-section rates. Their higher rates don't necessarily reflect the average patient's experience.) While hospitals are supposed to provide you with their C-section rates, you might have some trouble obtaining accurate information about the rates for individual physicians. Probably the best thing to do is to call around and talk to labor and delivery nurses. Of all people, they'll know which doctors have high C-section rates. Local childbirth educators and doulas can also be valuable sources for this information. (See Resources, page 197, for information about finding educators and doulas in your area.)

Up for Discussion

"You have to find a doctor who is really willing to work with you to avoid a cesarean," says Lani, 32, who was thwarted in her desire to attempt a vaginal birth after a cesarean by a change in hospital policy late in her pregnancy. "To a lot of doctors, I found, it's not important. They're there, they feel, just to protect your life." In other words, Lani says, these doctors jump more readily to the conclusion that a C-section is necessary to save the mother or the baby. They don't understand why women would care about the delivery process as long as it resulted in a healthy baby.

Lani practically took the words right out of the mouths of a research team from the University of Bristol in England, which recently published a small study of women who had either had an unplanned C-section or a vaginal delivery involving forceps or vacuum extraction. "It is essential that women are listened to if progress is to be made in the provision of safe and acceptable intrapartum (labor and delivery) care," the Bristol researchers wrote in *BMJ*, a British medical journal. "The priority for the obstetrician is safe delivery for mother and baby,

TALKING POINT

If you're looking for a doctor with a low C-section rate, survey labor and delivery nurses, local doulas, or childbirth educators.

and to a large extent this is achieved. Maternal satisfaction with the birth experience must now be addressed."

Open for Business 24/7

Try to find a doctor who delivers at a hospital that has obstetricians and anesthesiologists in labor and delivery 24 hours a day, 7 days a week. Some of the most outspoken critics of the rising U.S. C-section rate blame it on doctors' convenience, not medical necessity. While that may be a bit of a stretch, even doctors themselves admit they're not always crazy about sitting around for hours as a patient's labor drags on, especially if it's overnight. In such cases, a C-section begins to look pretty attractive. But if physicians aren't pressed for time, if they have to remain in the hospital even if no one is in labor, they do fewer cesareans. Round-the-clock in-house coverage is one reason academic medical centers—hospitals that have an obstetrics residency program and are affiliated with medical schools—tend to have lower C-section rates than community hospitals.

Even among doctors who aren't in a rush to get home to their family, some may be quicker than others to perform a cesarean because they think labor is progressing too slowly. Given just a little more time, vaginal delivery might have been possible, without compromising the baby's or the mom's health.

Words from the Wise

Consider having your baby at a teaching hospital, if possible. Academic medical centers have obstetricians and anesthesiologists on site at all times. Since they have to be there anyway, they're less likely to rush in and perform a C-section if labor drags on longer than expected.

Handy with Tools

Find a doctor who's willing to use forceps or vacuum extraction, which is rapidly becoming a lost art. Physicians adept at using those tools are dwindling in number because so-called operative vaginal deliveries have developed a bad reputation. True, in unskilled hands, operative deliveries with forceps or vacuum extraction can injure the mother or the baby. But skilled doctors can use those tools to get a baby out even more quickly than if they had performed a C-section. If a doctor doesn't feel comfortable performing operative deliveries, "that person is going to cut you and do a cesarean," says Mark Landon, M.D., vice chair of obstetrics and gynecology at The Ohio State University. Yet, some obstetrical residency programs don't even train doctors in how to use forceps or vacuum extraction, because older doctors got burned with malpractice suits when they used them. Even when residents do learn how to use those tools, they might never get a chance to keep up their skills if they practice at a hospital that discourages their use.

Mothers sometimes simply need a little assistance from forceps or vacuum extraction right at the end of a long labor. "I do it a lot for maternal exhaustion," says Dartmouth OB/GYN Michele Lauria, M.D. "Gentle forceps don't hurt the baby." A study of nearly 600,000 California births bears her out. Published in 1999, it concluded that difficult labor, not the tools used to assist delivery, is what can lead to problems in babies. No matter whether they

TALKING POINT

When quizzing potential doctors for prenatal care, ask whether they're comfortable using forceps or vacuum extraction. While you're at it, you might ask them how often they use those tools. That skill could mean the difference between a vaginal delivery and a C-section.

were delivered with the help of forceps, vacuum extraction, or an unplanned C-section, the risk of bleeding in the brain was half a percent, which is double that of babies delivered vaginally without any assistance. Often, such bleeding is minor, but it can cause serious complications.

Location, Location, Location

Another way to reduce your odds of having a C-section may be to avoid doctors and hospitals completely. That's not saying you should deliver at home alone. But a recent study found that prenatal care from certified nurse midwives in collaboration with obstetricians, coupled with access to a freestanding birthing center, significantly reduced women's chances of having a C-section. The researchers compared pregnant women who went to "collaborative care birth center" programs with those who went the more traditional route of an obstetrician and delivery in a hospital. (Although not covered in this study, many midwives practice in hospitals with special rooms, equipped with warm tubs, birth stools, rocking chairs, and non-hospital beds. If you're interested in this kind of arrangement, ask your midwife or check with the hospital to see if they have a similar facility.)

You might say, "Duh, of course women going to midwives are going to have fewer cesareans. Midwives don't do C-sections, so they attract the patients least likely to need one or want one. Obstetricians get the high-risk patients." And you'd have a good point. The only way researchers could be pretty sure they were comparing apples to apples—thus reducing the likelihood of biased results— would be if they randomly assigned pregnant women to either the obstetricians or the midwives. But, as you can imagine, researchers might have a hard time recruiting pregnant women for a study in which they didn't get to have a say in who cared for them or where they delivered. As an alternative, the San Diego Birth Center Study

Words from the Wise

If you're determined to deliver vaginally, find out whether there's a freestanding birthing center nearby where certified nurse midwives provide prenatal care in collaboration with obstetricians. Research suggests that such an arrangement can reduce your chance of having a cesarean delivery.

took great pains to ensure that the women who opted to go to the obstetrician were just as low-risk for a cesarean as those who chose to go to the midwifery practice. If they weren't, they were excluded from the study.

Even though no participant appeared likely to need a cesarean at the beginning of the study, a higher proportion of women under the obstetricians' care ended up delivering that way. After accounting for factors that could affect C-section risk, such as type and number of previous deliveries, researchers found that about 5 percent more of the women under an obstetrician's care delivered by cesarean. That may not sound like much, but it works out to C-section rates of roughly 16 percent in the traditional care group and 11 percent in the midwifery group.

DON'T BE SHY: LET YOUR DOCTOR KNOW WHAT YOU WANT

Okay. You've picked a doctor who seems to have a relatively low C-section rate. But no doctor is a mind reader. If you want to avoid a C-section, you've got to make it clear right from the beginning, like Barbara did. Tell your doctor you'd like her to do everything possible to avoid a cesarean. Ask her to note your wishes in your chart, in case she isn't on call when you're admitted to the hospital in labor, and if you have a birth plan (which should be no longer than one page) be sure to include that request.

Clearly, some C-sections are unavoidable, no matter how much you'd like to deliver vaginally. But simply making your wishes known could really make a difference if you fall into the gray area of cases—such as if your labor is progressing slowly—in which either a cesarean or a vaginal delivery is possible.

It helped that Barbara had a longstanding relationship with her obstetrician. Even a doctor whom you haven't known for a long time should be sympathetic to your desires, as long as you're not too dictatorial or unrealistic. No matter what you learn in your childbirth class or read in pregnancy books, forget about drawing up a lengthy, extremely detailed birth plan that covers everything from whether you want the lights on to what music should be played in the labor and delivery room. "It sometimes creates hostility right from the get-go," says Kaiser Permanente OB/GYN Bruce Flamm, M.D., of Riverside, California. "The nurses get very upset when somebody comes in with a 4-page birth plan. The doctor often gets very concerned when he sees a birth plan like that. Things tend to go from bad to worse."

Like most people, doctors aren't exactly keen on confrontation, and their distaste for it has grown along with their malpractice insurance premiums. These days, a more politic approach (that is, a relatively short summary of how you'd like labor and delivery to proceed) would serve you better. You don't have to walk on eggshells. Simply acknowledging that your doctor is the expert can make her more receptive to your wishes. If you've chosen your doctor well, you should feel comfortable deferring to her opinion should the need arise.

Not that you have to suffer in silence once you're admitted to the hospital. Go ahead and pack your iPod or Walkman and a selection of your favorite music to deliver by, whether it's Bruce Springsteen, Bach, or the Bulgarian State Female Television & Radio Women's Choir (really, their rendition of "Oh! Susannah" is amazing). In labor and delivery, certainly feel free to ask for whatever it takes to make you feel comfortable, whether it's an adjustment of the thermostat or a dip in a whirlpool, if it's available and you're not hooked up to an epidural. You just don't have to put every single request in writing.

And remember, even the best-laid plans can go awry, especially when the plans in question relate to a process as fluid, if you'll pardon the pun, as childbirth. "I did have this birth plan, natural this, natural that," recalls Joan. "I wrote mine and turned it in at about 6 months into my pregnancy. Still euphoric, still feeling great." Then she went a week past her due date. "I wanted it over with. I was like 'Sure, Pitocin, bring it on.' Then the contractions really started getting wickedly strong. By that time, I was about 5 centimeters dilated. I said, 'How much worse are these contractions going to get?'"

> ### Words from the Wise
>
> *A super-detailed birth plan could backfire. You certainly should tell your doctor if you'd like to avoid having a C-section, but you don't need to submit a play-by-play description of how you expect labor and delivery to pan out. You could even begin your plan by noting that it's not intended to be a script, but rather an opportunity for you to express your preferences and desires regarding your baby's birth.*

"A lot worse," her doctor told her. Bring on the painkiller, an intravenous narcotic. "It made my head very fuzzy, but the pain was very acute. This isn't doing the trick. My tolerance for pain was a lot less than I thought it would be." Bring on the epidural, which, thankfully, brought on some sleep. "They woke me up when I was at 10 centimeters," she recalls. After she had pushed for 4 hours, her doctor asked if she would mind if he used forceps to pull her stuck baby through the birth canal. "I was so exhausted. I said, 'Yeah, go ahead.' I kind of closed my eyes." Because of a rare, serious placenta complication that could recur, Joan, now 40, and her husband decided not to have any more children. But if they did, she knows that her birth plan would be short and to the point. "The birth plan that I made out, where I thought I could control the whole thing and knew how I would react at every moment, was just a crock," she says now. "If I did get pregnant again and wrote a birth plan, it would be one sentence: Just keep me and the baby alive."

Of course, your birth plan can be longer than a sentence, especially if it's your first baby and you and your OB/GYN are just getting to know each other. You have a head start if you've chosen a doctor you can trust, someone who shares your thoughts about childbirth. If you keep an open mind and focus on your ultimate goal—holding your healthy baby in your arms—you're likely to have a satisfying experience.

EATING FOR TWO:
DON'T BE POUND FOOLISH

Pregnancy may be the only time past puberty when you're actually expected to gain weight. But if you want to maximize your chances of having a vaginal delivery, you'll have to put down that donut and pick up your pace. Obesity before, as well as during, pregnancy appears to raise the likelihood that you'll deliver by C-section. And exercise during pregnancy can keep you in shape and help to limit your weight gain and your baby's, increasing the chance that you'll be able to deliver vaginally. Getting in shape for that athletic event called labor is one of the best ways you can minimize your chance of having a C-section.

Laura Riley, M.D., an obstetrician at Massachusetts General Hospital in Boston, can't understand how anyone could be surprised about the connection between obesity and cesareans. "I'm sort of tired of hearing that doctors want to do cesarean sections," says Riley, chair of the committee on obstetrics practice for the American College of Obstetricians and Gynecologists. "Well, guess what? Moms want to eat until they can't eat anymore." Generally, the more moms pack on the pounds, the bigger their babies are at birth, setting the stage for a C-section. "What do people expect?" says Riley. "You can't get a watermelon out of a very small spot. It seems like common sense to me."

Riley advises her patients not to gain more than 25 or 30 pounds during their pregnancy, plenty for growing a healthy 7- to 8-pound baby. "I'm not asking you to be on the cover of *Vogue*," she says. "People forget that this is a medical issue."

Probably only half of her patients pay any attention, though. As a result, 14 percent of the babies in her practice are macrosomic, which means they weigh more than 8 pounds, 12 ounces. (On the other hand, you don't want to gain too little weight, because that could increase your risk of delivering prematurely.)

The respected Institute of Medicine, part of the National Academy of Sciences in Washington, D.C., suggests that normal-weight women gain about 20 percent of their ideal pre-pregnancy body weight during pregnancy. The American College of Obstetricians and Gynecologists puts it a different way:

- If you're of normal weight, you should gain 25 to 35 pounds during your pregnancy.
- If you're underweight, you should gain 28 to 40 pounds.
- If you're overweight, you should gain only 15 to 25 pounds.
- If you're carrying twins, you get to gain 35 to 45 pounds.

In 2001, 12 percent of pregnant U.S. women gained more than 46 pounds, and it's likely the vast majority of them were neither underweight when they conceived, nor carrying twins.

Researchers from the National Center for Health Statistics recently explored whether the rise in the U.S. C-section rate through the 1990s paralleled an increase in excessive weight gains in mothers-to-be. They focused on first-time mothers who delivered a full-term, single baby.

Words from the Wise

Pregnancy is a great time to hone healthy eating habits. By cutting out empty calories—that is, fattening foods with little nutritional value—you're not only getting your baby off to a good start, but you're reducing your chance of needing a C-section.

Excessive weight gain was defined as more than 40 pounds.

From 1990 to 2000, the proportion of first-time moms who gained an excessive amount of weight rose from 19 percent to 24 percent. During that same time, women who gained more than 40 pounds accounted for an increasingly greater proportion of C-sections. By 2000, although they represented only about 24 percent of all first-time pregnant women, they accounted for 28 percent of all cesarean deliveries.

Interestingly, while pregnant women on average got bigger, their babies didn't. Among mothers who gained more than 40 pounds, the proportion of babies weighing more than 8¾ pounds actually fell by more than 19 percent. Apparently, bigger babies weren't the main factor behind the rise in C-section rates, the researchers concluded. Nonetheless, they note, there are more pregnant women than ever packing on excessive pounds, and they account for a growing proportion of cesarean deliveries.

Ideally, you should be at a normal weight when you conceive. Because no matter how little weight you gain while pregnant, if you're overweight from the beginning, research suggests you're at

Words from the Wise

If you're not pregnant yet but hope to be, try to slim down to your ideal weight before you conceive.

an increased risk of having a C-section. But if you're closer to a size 18 than a size 8, you're in good company. More than a third of U.S. women of childbearing age are overweight, and their numbers are increasing. Take Jefferson County, Alabama. The proportion of women in that county who weighed 200 or more pounds at their first prenatal visit jumped from just over 7 percent in 1980 to nearly 25 percent in 2000.

Being overweight not only increases your risk of complications like diabetes and high blood pressure that can lead to a C-section, but the extra pounds alone appear to raise your chances of having one. A University of Washington study suggests that even if you're fairly slender when you get pregnant, you're more likely to have a C-section than your really skinny friend. The risk of gestational diabetes, preeclampsia, cesarean delivery, and other complications begins rising once you hit a pre-pregnancy body mass index, or BMI, of 20, the study found. (And most women would kill for a BMI of 20). Usually, a normal BMI—a measure of weight for height—is considered to be 20 to 24.9, while overweight is 25 to 29.9 and obese is a 30 and over. (If you're 5-foot-4 and weighed 140 pounds when you got pregnant, for example, your BMI was 24. If you weighed only 116, your BMI was 20, lucky you.)

Even if you don't have diabetes or high blood pressure, the heavier you are when you conceive, the more likely you are to deliver by C-section, according to the University of Washington study. If your pre-pregnancy BMI falls within the normal range, you're still 30 percent more likely to deliver by C-section than underweight women (obviously, though, there are far better ways to reduce your risk of a cesarean than starving yourself!). If you're overweight when you get pregnant, your chance of delivering in the O.R. is about 80 percent higher than that of very lean woman. And if you're obese, your chance of having a cesarean delivery is nearly double that of an underweight woman.

New research by National Institutes of Health scientists provides one possible explanation as to why obese women are more likely to have a cesarean, even if they have no weight-related complications that might predispose them to one. The researchers found that before their cervix dilated to 6 centimeters, obese women had a significantly slower labor than normal weight women. For example, it took normal weight women an average of 86 minutes to progress from 3 centimeters to 4, but it took obese women an average of 125 minutes. More than half of the C-sections in obese women were performed before they reached 6 centimeters dilation, compared to only 40 percent of cesareans in normal weight women.

By the way, just because you were an enviable size 2 when you got pregnant doesn't mean you don't have to worry about how much weight you pack on. In fact, if you're that small to begin with, even the 25- to 30-pound weight gain that Laura Riley generally recommends to her patients might increase your chances of

TALKING POINT

If you are very overweight and hope to avoid a C-section, it's especially important to choose a patient doctor. That's because it might take you longer to dilate, at least in the beginning, than a woman who's at her ideal weight.

delivering by cesarean. A Yale University study of 2,301 women from the New Haven, Connecticut, area found that gaining more than 28 percent of your prepregnancy weight doubles your risk of having a C-section. Say you weighed 100 pounds before you conceived, and you've been chugalugging Dairy Queen Blizzards for their calcium content (yeah, right) ever since you saw that thin blue line on a home pregnancy test. Well, if those Blizzards snowball into a weight gain of more than 28 pounds, you've doubled your risk of having a C-section. Stick with nonfat or lowfat dairy products instead (or at least an occasional small DQ cone instead of a daily Blizzard) and you'll be doing yourself and your baby a favor.

AT YOUR SERVICE:
THINK ABOUT HIRING A DOULA

In the old days, when women gave birth at home, other women made sure that they were as comfortable as possible. Even today, when most births occur in the hospital, it's not uncommon for close female friends or relatives to accompany laboring women. But those friends or relatives usually are not healthcare professionals; and even if they are, they're probably not familiar with the hospital in question. So while they play an important role, they can't fully support the pregnant woman during labor. "They have an emotional bond with the woman, no question, but they're not prepared to deal with all the dynamics of labor or all the dynamics of the hospital," says Ellen Hodnett, a nursing professor at the University of Toronto. "It's an awful lot of a burden to put on somebody."

And you can't necessarily count on a nurse or a midwife to help you get the delivery you'd like. A midwife who's a hospital employee will be concerned about playing by the institution's rules, Hodnett says. She "has to be able to survive there beyond an individual woman's labor." Hodnett reached those conclusions after leading a study of nearly 7,000 pregnant women. When the moms-to-be were in labor, they were randomly assigned to receive either the usual care provided at their hospital, whatever that was, or continuous support—advice, information and comfort—by a specially trained nurse. Hodnett and her collaborators found no significant differences between the two groups or their babies. The C-section rates were nearly identical. The researchers suspect that the high rates of medical interventions such as C-sections in the participating hospitals overwhelmed any benefit from continuous labor support.

After combining the results of her research with 14 other similarly designed studies, Hodnett found that continuous support during labor from caregivers who were not hospital employees cut the risk of a C-section by just over a quarter. Labor support from non-hospital employees also reduced women's likelihood of requiring the assistance of vacuum extraction or forceps nearly by half. The benefit was greatest when the caregiver was an outsider present expressly to fill that role.

This is where specially trained women called doulas come in. Doula is a Greek word meaning "servant woman" or "handmaiden." You might also hear doulas referred to as labor or birth companions, labor or birth assistants, or labor support specialists. In North America, an estimated 35,000 people have received doula training. They typically charge between $200 and $800, which usually

Words from the Wise

Some hospitals have specially trained women called doulas on staff to support patients in labor. But research suggests that you'd be better off hiring a doula from outside the hospital. Check out the Web site for Doulas of North America (www.dona.org) to find names of doulas in your area.

covers at least one prenatal visit, labor and delivery, and a home visit after the birth. Not just any doula will do for any woman. "You've got to feel a good connection," Hodnett advises. "The relationship between the woman and the doula is critical. If you don't come away with a good feeling of comfort and trust, then it's not a good relationship."

When Susan L.'s doctor tried mightily to discourage her from attempting a VBAC, she decided to hire a doula. "I knew one other person who hired a doula because she wanted a VBAC," explains Susan, 41. She found a Web site that listed doulas in her state. "I just went through the list and called different ones and asked them about VBACs." Every one of them recommended she call Kim, who had a VBAC herself and had attended a number of them. Susan interviewed a few other doulas before hiring Kim for $400. "We had two prenatal visits. She came over, and we just talked about what my fears were, what I wanted for my birth, just got to know each other. The second visit, we did some relaxation, talked about what helps me relax, some music choices. Then I called her when I was in labor, and she came over. The great thing about her is she knew when it was time to go to the hospital." When Susan began hunkering down on her hands and knees instead of standing, Kim observed "she's getting close to the ground" and asked whether the car was packed to go to the hospital. "Then my water broke. I went into active labor at that point. I couldn't have done it naturally without her. I think I would have gotten an epidural." (For more information about VBACs, see chapter 6, "Once a Cesarean, Always a Cesarean?," page 158.)

Susan had delivered her first child, a son now 21 months old, by a C-section because her doctor felt her labor wasn't moving along

Words from the Wise

Hoping to have a VBAC? Look for a doula who has experience with such deliveries.

quickly enough. She blames the fact she was tethered to a fetal monitor and couldn't get out of bed and move around. Kim had a plan to deal with that situation should it arise. "If they were going to make me stay in bed, she knew how to get me moving in different positions that would help facilitate the natural thing," Susan recalls. Fortunately, the hospital at which she delivered her second child had telemetry, which uses radio waves to transmit the baby's heart tones to the nurses' station. Susan could walk, squat, keep moving. "Things went faster the second time." Her water broke at 11:30 A.M., and her 8 pound, 10½ ounce daughter was born at 7:30 P.M. Along with Kim, Susan had two friends, her sister, and her husband lending moral support. "It was just the most perfect birth," Susan says. "I couldn't have asked for anything better."

If you're thinking about hiring a doula for your labor and delivery, Doulas of North America (DONA), a professional organization, suggests that you ask candidates about more than just their fees and training (although those are important, too). Some key questions for your potential doula:

- What is your philosophy about childbirth and supporting women and their partners during labor?
- Will you meet with me beforehand to discuss your role in supporting me during childbirth?
- Can I call you with questions or concerns before and after the birth?

Juliet, 33, credits a doula with helping her succeed in her attempt for a VBAC. Pregnant with her second child, Juliet didn't want a repeat of her first delivery, a C-section performed when the baby's head could already be seen through her vagina. Although she switched doctors, she still planned to deliver at the same hospital where she had her first daughter, now 3 years old. Her new doctor wasn't on call when she went into labor, but she had the same labor nurse as when she had her C-section. And that nurse wasn't a fan of VBACs. She told Juliet that she had to stay in bed on continuous monitoring—not exactly what Juliet had planned. For her second delivery, though, Juliet had hired a doula, who successfully ran interference for her. Juliet could walk around, take showers, do whatever she needed to, as long as her baby's heart rate was checked every 20 minutes.

MOTHER NATURE USUALLY KNOWS BEST: TRY NOT TO JUMP-START LABOR BY GETTING INDUCED

If you're 2 weeks past your due date and you feel like you're heading toward a record for the world's longest gestation, induction—in which drugs are used to bring on labor—can be a good thing. Your uterus might not be what it used to be in the earlier months of your pregnancy. Your amniotic fluid might be drying up and your placenta might be disintegrating. Time to get that baby out, pronto—and having your labor induced could help you deliver vaginally. It's also time to move things along if you or your baby is sick and delivery must be expedited, if your bag of waters breaks and labor doesn't begin, or if you have a uterine infection.

But what if you're only at 38 or 39 weeks and simply sick of being pregnant (it happens sometimes), or hoping to deliver before your doctor goes on vacation? If you're a healthy first-time mom about to deliver a full-term (37 weeks to 40 weeks) baby, labor induction nearly doubles your risk of a C-section, from just under 14 percent to just under 25 percent, according to a recent Harvard study. And remember those National Institutes of Health researchers who observed that labor progresses more slowly in obese patients? They found a similar situation in women whose labor had been induced and cervix "ripened" (softened with medication or pressure from a special balloon device to prepare it for dilation).

Apparently, if your body isn't ready to give birth, trying to induce labor might be like trying to start a campfire with wet wood and some

Words from the Wise

No matter how appealing it might sound to schedule when you're going into labor, remember that getting induced can nearly double your chance of having a C-section.

matches. Even if you manage to spark contractions, they might not be effective in pushing that baby out—setting you up for an unplanned cesarean. And another thing: While generally considered to be safe, induction can also increase your risk of uterine rupture, especially if drugs called prostaglandins are used and you've had a prior C-section.

Despite concerns about the rising cesarean delivery rate, induction of labor has become one of the fastest-growing medical procedures in the United States. From 1989 (the year birth certificates began requiring information about the practice) to 1998, the proportion of U.S. births in which labor was induced more than doubled, from 9 percent to 19.2 percent. The 1998 rate was even higher for non-Hispanic white women—nearly 23 percent. In 2001, the nationwide labor induction rate climbed to 20.5 percent, an all-time high. If the pace continues—and there's no reason to think it won't—the U.S. labor induction rate will hit 30 percent by 2007, according to one estimate. If you excluded women who've scheduled a C-section and, therefore, aren't candidates for induction, the rate would be much higher.

One explanation for the rising rates is that doctors are better equipped to detect problems that could endanger pregnancies, such

Looking Back

Not until the early 19th century did Dr. James Barry become the first doctor in the British Empire to perform a cesarean in which both mother and child survived. Dr. Barry was one talented individual. Barry qualified as a doctor of medicine by age 17 and performed that successful C-section sometime in his twenties. About a century later, a grandson of the baby who survived a cesarean delivery became the prime minister of South Africa in 1924. But the most amazing part of this story is that James Barry was actually a woman. Now recognized as the first British woman physician, Barry had successfully masqueraded as a man from 1809—the year she entered Edinburgh University—until her death in 1865. During her lifetime, most medical schools wouldn't admit women. Barry recognized at an early age that her only chance to succeed as a physician in 19th century Britain was as a man.

as borderline high blood pressure or an abnormally low level of amniotic fluid. Another contributing factor: Increasing numbers of women with chronic diseases (such as heart ailments) that could complicate pregnancies, are having babies.

But let's face it. There aren't that many more women or babies whose poor health requires a speedy delivery. And the number of women waddling past the midpoint of their 10th month of pregnancy hasn't increased dramatically. If a growing number of problem pregnancies was the sole reason for the soaring induction rate, you'd have to feel pretty sorry for the women of Wisconsin. In 1998, pregnant women in that state were nearly four times more likely to be induced than their counterparts in Hawaii.

"Psychosocial indications" such as convenience have become a common reason for elective labor inductions. Think about one other obvious difference between Wisconsin and Hawaii. The weather, of course.

Imagine that you live in Milwaukee and that you're due to deliver in late January, just when a snowstorm is expected to hit. The thought of scheduling an induction before the roads become impassable is pretty appealing.

When government researchers examined 1998 birth certificates, they found mention of a medical reason for only about a quarter of full-term babies whose delivery was induced. It's possible that the medical indication simply wasn't noted on the birth certificate, but the finding does suggest that a large number of labor inductions aren't medically necessary. In some institutions, as many as half of all inductions are elective. They represent 10 percent of all births, not counting repeat C-sections. While hospitals usually track doctors' C-section rates, they don't pay that much attention to induction rates. But in some hospitals, such as Brigham and Women's Hospital and Beth Israel Deaconess Medical Center in Boston, doctors are forbidden to induce labor without a medical reason before the 39th week of the pregnancy.

Although labor induction may appear to be more convenient, doctors should inform patients that it frequently leads to a longer labor and a longer hospital stay, notes Kathleen Rice Simpson, a perinatal clinical nurse specialist in St. Louis who recently wrote a review on the subject. "The issue of convenience is not well understood, and often that convenience is for the benefit of the healthcare

TALKING POINT

When choosing an OB/GYN, ask about labor induction rates. The more women a doctor induces, the more C-sections he's likely to perform.

provider rather than for the mother and her baby," Simpson says. "I'm not against all elective inductions. I just think women should be fully informed of the implications." If they are fully informed, they just might reconsider their desire to be induced.

As a family physician, Ellen is well aware that inducing labor too early in a healthy first-time mom raises her C-section risk. But she agreed to take a chance with an elective induction because she very much wanted her obstetrician to be present when she delivered her firstborn. He'd been so supportive when she previously had a miscarriage.

Ellen's doctor scheduled her induction a week and a half before her due date. He couldn't wait any longer, because he was scheduled to undergo surgery for carpal tunnel syndrome. "I was leaving it up to him. I really had a lot of confidence in this doctor, because I'd already had a miscarriage," she says. Shortly after she was induced, her water broke. "I wasn't anywhere near ready to have a baby, basically. I went along with it. I was certainly educated enough to know there was going to be a risk of a C-section. But then once my water broke, I knew I was going to have a baby one way or another."

Sure enough, Ellen delivered her first daughter, now 10, by C-section after many hours of labor during which her cervix failed to fully dilate. The night after she delivered, she couldn't help but overhear the conversation about her at the nearby nurses' station. "I could hear them saying, 'She deserved a C-section. If she's going to be induced a week and a half early, what does she expect?'"

The nurses had a point, although they didn't have to be so snippy about it, especially within earshot of Ellen. You can't blame her for wanting to have her trusted doctor deliver her baby. But she took a gamble on induction that didn't quite pan out the way she had hoped—except for the part about her healthy, beautiful daughter.

PAIN, NO GAIN: GO AHEAD AND GET THAT EPIDURAL IF YOU WANT IT

You might have heard that getting an epidural will increase your chances of having a C-section. Studies in which researchers compared women who chose to get an epidural with those who didn't found that the former group was about four times more likely to need a cesarean, forceps, or vacuum extraction than the latter group. That seems to make sense. After all, more than half of the pregnant women in the United States receive epidural analgesia to relieve labor pain, and the country's C-section rate is at an all-time high. Epidurals are first-rate painkillers, but if you can't feel anything down below, how are you supposed to push that baby out, right?

Maybe, maybe not. Studies that randomly assigned women to an epidural or to another form of painkiller have had mixed results. Some found that epidurals given before the cervix was dilated to 5 centimeters increased the risk of a cesarean delivery by 50 percent. Other studies found epidurals didn't raise the C-section risk. But a review that pooled the results of 11 randomized trials comparing epidurals with other painkillers or none at all found epidurals had no effect on cesarean rates.

Still, when an American College of Obstetricians and Gynecologists' task force looked for ways to lower the U.S. C-section rate, it recommended that, when feasible, doctors use another painkiller in first-time mothers until they were 4 or 5 centimeters dilated. Some hospitals went overboard, though. They began withholding epidurals from all patients until they reached that magic 4 or 5 centimeters of dilation. So ACOG and the American Society of Anesthesiologists issued a joint opinion on the matter: "There is no other circumstance where it is considered acceptable for a person to experience untreated severe pain, amenable to safe intervention, while under a physician's care." If a patient wants an epidural, she

Words from the Wise

You can have your epidural and deliver vaginally, too. Just keep in mind that it might slow things down a bit. If you want to delay getting an epidural, narcotic painkillers can provide relief.

should get it, as long as there's no medical reason for her not to have one, the statement concludes.

Even so, Dartmouth's Lauria, speaking from both personal and professional experience, suggests that you try to hold off on getting an epidural until you're 4 or 5 centimeters dilated or until your baby is low in your pelvis—although, she acknowledges, there aren't a lot of data to support her recommendation. Until you're that far along in labor, narcotic painkillers, such as Demerol, can take the edge off. Lauria is only 5-foot-2 and 105 pounds, but she pushed each of her three children out in 10 minutes and had an epidural every time. Kathryn, 41, swears that her first three children ended up being delivered by C-section because she got an epidural too soon. With her next four children, she waited until her cervix was dilated to 6 or 7 centimeters, instead of 4, and the baby had moved low in her pelvis. And she delivered vaginally every time.

Women who get an epidural may indeed be more likely to have a cesarean than women who don't, but don't blame the epidural, says Jun Zhang, Ph.D., a medical epidemiologist at the National Institute for Child Health and Human Development, part of the National Institutes of Health. Other than the epidural itself, there's another big difference between women who get one and women who don't. Think about what motivates women to ask for an epidural. Pain, of course. Well, women whose labor isn't progressing normally may be quicker to ask for an epidural than women whose labor is progressing smoothly, says Zhang, who co-authored the study about whether epidurals increased C-section risk. And, naturally, women whose labor isn't progressing smoothly are more likely to end up having a C-section.

Several studies have found that women whose babies are facing their stomach instead of their back—a position that greatly increases the chance of a C-section (read more about the occiput posterior position in chapter 1, page 19)—are more likely to get epidurals than women whose babies are facing their back, the normal position for delivery. But further research is needed to determine whether epidurals increase the risk of a sunny-side up baby or whether women whose babies are in this position are more likely to ask for an epidural because their labor is so painful. ("Back labor" can be especially trying because your baby's skull and spine, rather than his soft face and tummy, are pressed against your sensitive back.)

You don't get off totally scot-free if you choose to get an epidural. Some studies have found that epidurals prolong both the first phase of labor, when your cervix is dilating, and the second, when you're pushing. Zhang's study found that it didn't take any longer for the cervix to become fully dilated, but women who received epidurals had to push an average of 25 minutes longer than women who didn't. If you and your doctor don't consider that epidurals can prolong labor, it's possible you could end up with a C-section.

In at least one respect, Zhang says, epidurals might actually prove to be advantageous. His research found that doctors weren't as hasty to use forceps or vacuum extraction to help babies through the birth canal in patients who'd had an epidural. That's probably because the women weren't complaining about the pain of pushing as much as those delivering au naturel. So when doctors finally decided to use the instruments with patients who had an epidural, babies tended to be lower in the birth canal than in those women who didn't have an epidural. When babies are lower in the birth canal, doctors don't have to use as much force to extract them, minimizing the risk of injuries.

If you're worried about the effect of an epidural on your baby, a recent report by anesthesiologists at the University of Tennessee Health Sciences Center should help put your mind at ease. Most anesthetics and painkillers currently in use cross into the placenta when given to pregnant women. But, if used appropriately, they're well-tolerated by the baby. Epidurals actually improve the flow of oxygen and blood to the placenta, which could be especially helpful to the baby if mom has pregnancy-induced high blood pressure, according to the researchers.

TAKE YOUR TIME:
IN LABOR, PATIENCE IS A VIRTUE

While you don't want to give birth in your car on your way to the hospital, it's not a good idea to head there as soon as you feel your first contraction. If you're trying to avoid a C-section, "wait until labor is really established before you come into the hospital," says Eugene Declercq, professor of maternal and child health at Boston University. "If you're in the hospital and labor stops and they give you the option to go home, go home. If you stay in the hospital, you'll be a high-risk case." The first—or latent—phase of labor can last for days. "If you're there early in labor, there's this feeling: 'She's been here a long time. We have to do something,' " Hodnett says. "There's a lot of 'Well, she's here, let's induce her.' " And we know what can happen next.

So how do you know when you should go to the hospital? The first step usually is to call your doctor or midwife. Call immediately if any of the following apply:

• You think your bag of waters broke.
• Your contractions are regular and 5 minutes apart.
• Your baby is suddenly moving more or less than before.

When your contractions become stronger and more frequent no matter whether you're lying down or standing, it's probably time to go to the hospital. Even if you're truly in labor when you arrive at the hospital, don't be disappointed if many hours pass before you get to greet your new baby. Meanwhile, keep yourself well-hydrated by drinking plenty of fluids in early labor and sucking on ice chips during labor (don't forget to urinate when you feel the urge). Birthing a baby, especially a first baby, usually is long, hard work, and any woman who thinks otherwise is fooling herself. Unrealistic notions about childbirth may increase your chances of ending up with C-section.

Words from the Wise

You may have heard about women who gave birth in a hospital hallway on their way to labor and delivery, or even in their car on their way to the hospital. Forget about them. It's perfectly normal to labor hours and hours before giving birth, especially if you're a first-timer. If you steel yourself for a long labor, you—and your doctor— will be less likely to grow impatient and rush to a C-section. You could even end up being pleasantly surprised.

"In some ways, it's an expectation issue," Zhang says. "If you expect the labor is going to be long, probably you just let it go longer. You're less anxious." But if you panic because things aren't moving along as quickly as you thought they would, you could be setting yourself up to have a cesarean birth.

A BABY IN DISTRESS:
THE CHALLENGE OF INTERPRETING
ELECTRONIC FETAL MONITORING

Chances are you'll be hooked up to a fetal monitor when you go into labor, but be prepared for false alarms that can increase your risk of a C-section. Electronic fetal monitoring is used during labor and delivery in 85 percent of U.S. pregnancies. Usually, a belt or a stretchy fabric girdle is strapped around the mother's abdomen to hold ultrasound sensors in place. Babies' heart rates normally drop during a contraction and then come back up to speed afterward. A drastic drop in heart rate during a contraction or a delay in getting back to normal afterward could be a sign that the baby isn't getting enough oxygen. This is commonly referred to as "fetal distress."

Most experts would agree that fetal monitoring is essential in certain cases. If you're trying to deliver vaginally after a prior C-section, or if your labor is induced or begins too early, your baby should be monitored. That's also holds true if your baby is in the breech position or appears to be small considering how far along you are in your pregnancy.

But, of course, such cases represent far fewer than 85 percent of pregnancies. That's the problem. Despite the wide use of electronic fetal monitoring, study after study has found it provides no benefit in the majority of pregnancies, those low-risk cases in which complications are unlikely. More than 18,000 women participated in studies in which they were randomly assigned to receive either electronic fetal monitoring or periodic checking of the baby's heart rate with a stethoscope or similar device. Babies whose mothers were tethered to electronic fetal monitors were no less likely to experience dire outcomes, such as cerebral palsy, score low on the Apgar test, require intensive care, or die. But they were about 40 percent more likely to be delivered by cesarean section. Not surprisingly, as the use of electronic fetal monitoring has grown, so has the country's C-section rate.

When fetal monitoring is used routinely, it triggers a lot of false alarms. Sometimes, simply turning from your back onto your side can transform what appears to be a baby in distress into one whose heart is doing just fine, thank you. In fact, back in 1988, the American College of Obstetricians and Gynecologists (ACOG) deemed the term "fetal distress" misleading and recommended abandoning it. In light of the randomized studies' results, ACOG concluded that periodically checking the baby's heart rate is an acceptable alternative to continuous electronic fetal monitoring. If, like most women's, yours is a low-risk pregnancy, ACOG recommends that your doctor check your baby's heart rate at least every half hour in the first stage of labor and at least every 15 minutes in the second, or pushing stage. If your pregnancy is high-risk, you need more frequent monitoring, but not necessarily continuous. Your doctor or nurse should check your baby's heart rate at least every 15 minutes in the first stage and at least every 5 minutes in the second stage, according to ACOG.

Researchers aren't sure why electronic fetal monitoring seems to increase your risk of having a cesarean section. They have some ideas, though. For one thing, when you're hooked up to an electronic fetal monitor, you're basically stuck in bed and can't walk around. Walking is thought to speed labor (although not every study has found that to be the case). For another thing, interpreting the peaks and valleys on those long paper monitoring strips can be pretty tricky. "There's a huge gray zone where we don't really have adequate understanding of what those tracings mean," says Catherine Spong, M.D., head of perinatology research at the National Institute of Child Health and Human Development.

One finding from the San Diego Birth Center Study illustrates the wide difference of opinion in interpreting those monitoring strip squiggles. If you'd received care at a prenatal clinic staffed by midwives and obstetricians, you had only a one in nine chance of hearing that your baby's heart rate was abnormal. If you'd received traditional care from an obstetrician, though, your chance of being told that your baby was in distress was one in five. Boston University's Declercq notes that diagnoses of fetal distress appear to peak in the late afternoon, suggesting that it's a convenient excuse for doctors to perform a C-section so they can get home to dinner. As you can imagine, if your doctor told you that your baby's tracings were worrisome, a cesarean delivery would begin to look pretty good.

Megan, 30, had planned to deliver vaginally at a birth center birth but ended up with a cesarean in the hospital. She places at least part of the blame on fetal monitoring. In the womb, her son had been facing her belly instead of her back, which made for a prolonged labor. She was given an epidural and Pitocin to speed up contractions. But then the fetal monitor showed that her baby's heart rate was dropping. So even though she had dilated to 8 centimeters, her doctor urged that she have a C-section. "It just kind of went from bad to worse," she now says. "They pretty much told my husband where to stand. He couldn't see anything. They were just very medically oriented." Megan herself didn't get to see the baby until several hours after his birth. Afterward, Megan, a physical therapist, looked at the tracings from the fetal monitor. She thought they showed that her son's heart rate always came back up quickly after the times that it slowed down.

TALKING POINT

Ask your doctor whether you can forego continuous fetal monitoring, which has been linked to an increased risk of having a C-section.

You should certainly ask about not having continuous monitoring, but you should understand that sometimes it's the only way that a labor and delivery nurse can keep track of more than one patient at a time. Even so, you should make your wishes known, because you might at least be able to reach a compromise of, say, 15 minutes of monitoring every hour. At the very least, find out whether the hospital where you expect to deliver uses telemetry. This type of fetal monitoring uses radio waves from a transmitter strapped to your thigh to send your baby's heart tones to the nurses' station. While telemetry doesn't eliminate the problem of false alarms, it does at least allow you to move around while being continuously monitored.

You can't know for sure whether you'll be able to deliver vaginally until you actually do it. But you can make choices that will increase your chances.

CHAPTER 6

ONCE A CESAREAN, ALWAYS A CESAREAN?

Sorting through the VBAC controversy

Ginger, 24, developed preeclampsia when pregnant with her first daughter and underwent an emergency C-section at 35 weeks. When she became pregnant again 2 years later, "I didn't even give it a second thought. I pretty much thought that I had to have another C-section," she recalls. "I felt disappointed. I'm just never going to have a baby normally."

Then a friend told her about vaginal birth after cesarean section, or VBAC. "I'd never even heard the term VBAC before. She kind of got me on the right path. I went back to my original doctor. He said, 'Yeah, we can totally do a VBAC, that's great.'"

By her next appointment, though, he'd had a change of heart. "Basically, what he told me is you get all stretched out, sex isn't that good, you have all these bladder problems. I was floored when I left his office, because I was excited about it. I was excited about trying for a VBAC. I needed somebody who's behind me 100 percent. I thought about doing a midwife, but because my insurance didn't cover it, I wasn't going to do it."

Instead, she asked midwives for names of VBAC-

*friendly doctors. She scheduled an appointment with one.
"He had a really good attitude about VBACs. He told me a
bunch of success stories. But there was an issue with the hospital there."*

*By her third appointment, he told her he expected lia-
bility concerns were going to force his hospital to ban VBACs
before her due date. Ginger was discouraged, but she held fast
to the idea of trying for a vaginal delivery. "I was almost in
my third trimester. I was getting close, and I didn't have a
real doctor yet."*

*This time, Ginger decided to pick the hospital first, then
the doctor. She focused on a teaching hospital that didn't have
a policy against VBACs. "I called the hospital, and I talked
to the nurses in the maternity ward and said, 'Who do you
guys like?'" Two different nurses on 2 different days named
the same doctor. "I went and interviewed him. When I came
in and talked to him, kind of gave him my history with my
first delivery, he didn't have any problems. He didn't think
my first C-section was necessary. That floored me. He said
they should have made more attempts at other things."*

*Ginger didn't go into labor until 5 days past her due
date. She arrived at the hospital at 6:00 A.M. and, after getting an epidural, delivered her second daughter at 1:58 P.M.
"She's just going to come right out, like toothpaste out of a
tube," Ginger's doctor had assured her. Turns out he was
right. "It was so easy at the end. I couldn't believe it."*

The main reason women schedule C-sections is because
they've previously had one. But just because you've had one
C-section (or more) doesn't mean you're destined to deliver all of
your subsequent babies that way. Like Ginger, maybe you'd like
the experience of delivering vaginally. Or perhaps the driving

reason behind your desire for a VBAC is the prospect of a shorter recovery time after delivery. After all, you'll now have at least one other child to care for besides your newborn (and we're not talking about your husband).

But maybe you've heard that VBACs can be dangerous. Maybe the hospital at which you were planning to deliver won't even let you try one. That's because a prior C-section does increase your risk of experiencing a uterine tear, or rupture, from the stress of contractions. Scheduling a repeat cesarean before labor begins will lower the chance that your uterus will rupture when you deliver. While uterine rupture sounds pretty scary, you have to keep in mind that the likelihood of one harming you or your baby is exceedingly small. For many women, the risks of undergoing a C-section, such as a greater chance of infection in moms or breathing problems in babies, outweigh those of attempting a VBAC.

THROUGH THE YEARS:
A BRIEF HISTORY OF VBACs

Way back in 1916, New York physician Edwin Cragin, M.D., presented a talk entitled "Conservatism in Obstetrics" to the Eastern Medical Society of the City of New York. He called for his colleagues to be conservative in their use of cesarean sections. Because no matter how carefully the uterine incision is stitched up, Cragin cautioned, you can never be sure whether it will withstand a subsequent pregnancy and labor without tearing, an accident that could have grave consequences for both mother and child. "This means the usual rule is once a cesarean, always a cesarean," he told his colleagues. But if doctors avoided performing C-sections in the first place—and in Cragin's time the rate was less than a tenth of what it is today—they wouldn't have to worry about uterine scars the next time their patients became pregnant.

Obstetricians followed Cragin's dictum for decades. As recently as 1970, basically all U.S. hospitals banned VBACs. Once a woman delivered by cesarean, all her subsequent deliveries had to be by cesarean. Later in the 1970s, though, some women began demanding the chance to deliver vaginally after a cesarean. They believed that the benefits of VBAC—including a shorter hospital stay and recovery and lower risks of infection and blood transfusion in mom and breathing problems in baby—outweighed the risks of a uterine rupture.

Their success impressed a panel of experts convened by the National Institutes of Health in 1981. The NIH had asked the panel to come up with ways to reign in the country's C-section rate, which had quadrupled between 1970 and 1980. Repeat cesarean delivery was one of the leading contributors to the ballooning U.S. C-section rate. So one of the NIH panel's main recommendations was that women with a prior C-section attempt a VBAC. At the time, only about 3 percent of candidate patients had successful VBACs, so, in the eyes of the panelists, there was a lot of room for improvement.

Despite the NIH experts' recommendation, interest in VBACs grew little through the 1980s. From 1980 through 1985, only 5 percent of women who'd previously had a C-section delivered their next baby vaginally. More than half a million of the repeat cesareans performed during that period could have been VBACs, government researchers estimated. In 1988, the U.S. C-section rate hit an all-time high (up until then) of 23 percent. A third of those cesareans were preplanned operations in women who'd had at least one previously.

Experts were concerned. C-sections cost more than vaginal deliveries, both in terms of the mother's recovery and in healthcare resources. But instead of trying to lower the C-section rate in women who'd never had one, insurers focused on preventing repeat cesareans. "The managed-care companies started mandating that you had to have a VBAC," says Dartmouth's Lauria. "You didn't have any choice." If you didn't try, some insurers wouldn't cover your elective C-section. The proportion of women with a prior cesarean who delivered vaginally increased steadily from 1989 to 1996, when it peaked at 28 percent.

For the most part, health plans were well-intentioned, Lauria says, but they overlooked an important fact: Not every woman is a good candidate for a VBAC. As more VBACs took place, of course, the U.S. C-section rate fell. But, at least in part because VBACs were being performed indiscriminately, uterine ruptures did occur, giving rise to a slew of medical malpractice suits. In 1997, for example, the County of Los Angeles paid $24 million to settle 49 claims related to VBACs at the University of Southern California Medical Center, according to the *Los Angeles Times*. That hospital had required VBACs on the grounds that they cost $2,300 less than elective repeat cesareans. It abandoned the policy in 1995 and left the decision about whether to attempt a VBAC up to the patient.

Huge awards for uterine rupture caused many medical malpractice insurers to raise their annual premiums for privately insured doctors who performed VBACs, sometimes by tens of thousands of dollars. The VBAC rate began to fall. Revised guidelines from the American College of Obstetricians and Gynecologists in 1999 helped fuel the decline. Probably the most controversial change in the new guidelines was a single word: "VBAC should be attempted in institutions equipped to respond to emergencies with physicians *immediately* available to provide emergency care." Previously, the obstetricians and gynecologists group had said that a surgical team should be "*readily* available," which had been interpreted to mean 30 minutes from the hospital.

A July 5, 2001, editorial in the *New England Journal of Medi-*

cine was the clincher. Harvard OB/GYN Michael Greene, M.D., wrote the piece in response to a controversial University of Washington study about VBACs and uterine rupture. The study found that women who attempted VBACs were three times more likely to experience a uterine rupture than women who had a planned C-section instead. Critics, and there have been many, argue that the Washington researchers couldn't possibly be sure that what they counted as a rupture really was. They had based their study on birth certificate information and hospital discharge data, both of which are notoriously inaccurate. Those concerns didn't stop Greene. "After a thorough discussion of the risks and benefits of attempting a vaginal delivery after cesarean section, a patient might ask, 'but doctor, what is the safest thing for my baby?'" Greene wrote. Given the study's findings, he wrote, "my unequivocal answer is: elective repeated cesarean section."

So for a variety of reasons, the proverbial pendulum began to swing too far the other way. From 1996 to 2002, the U.S. VBAC rate dropped by more than 50 percent, from a peak of 28 percent to just below 13 percent. That's only about a third of government experts' goal of a 37 percent VBAC rate by 2010.

Many hospitals thought the newly revised VBAC guidelines required that they have an obstetrician and anesthesiologist on hand 24 hours a day, 7 days a week. Rather than deal with the expense of increased staffing, some community hospitals, especially in rural areas, got out of the VBAC business entirely. Instead of requiring all women with a previous C-section to attempt a vaginal delivery, these hospitals began forcing them to have an elective repeat cesarean. "I don't think that was ACOG's intent when they published the guidelines," says Kaiser-Permanente OB/GYN Bruce Flamm, M.D., who practices in Riverside, California. "Their intent was to protect mothers and babies." Flamm thinks there's a way to comply with the ACOG guidelines without restricting women's access to

VBACs. In communities that have several hospitals with maternity units, the one that has in-house medical staff could do all the VBACs in town. Even in places with only one hospital, Flamm says, an obstetrician and anesthesiologist would have to spend the night only when a woman was attempting a VBAC, which wouldn't happen every night.

POWER PLAY: WHEN HOSPITALS BAN VBACs

Just as forcing all pregnant women with a prior C-section to attempt a VBAC is misguided, so is forcing all of them to have a repeat cesarean. The appropriate approach is somewhere in between. "There are candidates who should probably never VBAC because the risk is just too high, and there are those where it would be a crime not to let them VBAC," says Carolyn Zelop, M.D., associate professor of obstetrics and gynecology at the University of Connecticut. Your doctors needs to fully inform you of VBAC's risks and then let you decide whether it's worth it, says Mark Landon, M.D., vice chair of obstetrics and gynecology at The Ohio State University. Yes, there may be some risk involved, he says, but it's a definable risk. "It just becomes a matter of whether a woman is counseled well and is willing to assume that risk. For physicians and healthcare providers to deny women that option is, in my opinion, limiting their choices unnecessarily," says Landon.

But growing numbers of women are encountering hospital-wide VBAC bans. If you live in southern New Mexico, forget about finding a local hospital that will let you attempt a VBAC, says University of New Mexico family doctor Laurence Leeman, M.D. You might have a little more luck in New Hampshire or Vermont, says Lauria, but you'll still find that half the hospitals in those states will make you schedule a repeat cesarean. "I know of many women who have labored in parking lots, who are trying to do home

VBACs," she says. "Women who have had a prior section and then maybe two or three successful VBACs are being told they can't have a VBAC."

Lani, 32, was forced to deliver her second daughter by C-section because the hospital at which she was planning to give birth banned VBACs late in her pregnancy. Unlike some women, she couldn't switch hospitals because of insurance issues.

When Lani delivered her firstborn by C-section nearly 5 years ago, her doctor had assured her she was a prime candidate for a VBAC if she became pregnant again. Lani says her eldest "was just slightly crooked" in her womb: "They said she was trying to come out ear first." She was actually relieved when her doctor decided to do a C-section after 24 hours of labor, the last half of which involved 9-minute-long contractions. "I knew nothing but pain, so whatever they wanted to do was fine. After that labor, it was like, 'Yeah, whatever,'" she says. Besides ending her painful labor, Lani's cesarean had one other advantage: "I got an extra 2 weeks off work."

But when Lani became pregnant again, she hoped to deliver

TALKING POINT

If you want to try for a VBAC, make sure you deliver at a hospital that supports them. While a few states provide individual hospitals' VBAC rates (the proportion of women with a prior C-section who deliver vaginally), you might have to do some digging. One good source of information: nurses who work in the maternity units of local hospitals.

vaginally. Recovery from her first C-section was long, and it hurt. In her second pregnancy, her daughter was head-down very early and never moved from that position. "I was a little bit older, wiser, not as afraid of delivery," Lani recalls. "I think fear is a huge barrier to delivering naturally."

At a prenatal visit when she was 7 months pregnant, though, Lani learned she'd have to switch doctors and hospitals if she wanted to attempt a VBAC. Turns out none of the hospitals in her central California county (Lodi) would let women try VBACs. Her health insurance coverage wouldn't let her deliver in another county. "At that point I finally found out what it was all about. It was about the hospital's liability insurance. The hospital's liability insurance had mandated this," she says.

Lani's last battle was over when to schedule her C-section, and unfortunately, she lost that one, too. Her doctor wanted to schedule it 11 days before her due date, which was just too early in Lani's estimation. "It's not healthy for the baby. It's just convenient for the doctors," she says. "I told them I wanted to postpone it." Out of sheer frustration, she cried, but even her tears did not sway her doctor.

Her daughter was fine, although Lani still wishes the baby could have spent a little more time "wombing-in." As for Lani, she ended up spending a night in the intensive care unit after the delivery. She'd had a reaction to the morphine she'd been given to dull the pain after the operation.

Lauria finds it ironic that the same doctors who believe you have the right to choose a medically unnecessary C-section are restricting your choice of delivery after a prior cesarean. "I think VBAC is a woman's choice," she says. "It should be put in their hands, and not in the hands of hospital administrators and not in the hands of medical malpractice insurers. I think it's very paternalistic that it's been taken out of their hands."

Even if the hospitals in your immediate area haven't totally banned VBACs, you might find some a lot more open to them than others. It's not a black-and-white issue—once you confirm that a hospital allows VBACs, you have to find out what proportion of candidates actually attempt them. In a recent study of 17 U.S. hospitals, researchers found that the attempted VBAC rate ranged from 38 to 65 percent among women who were possible candidates. And, contrary to what happened in Lani's case, the difference here wasn't geographic. Their VBAC attempt rates may have been all over the map, but the 17 hospitals weren't: All but one of the hospitals in the study were within a 35-minute drive from the others. "VBAC rates varied drastically even for hospitals within 10 minutes of each other," says lead author George Macones, M.D., an OB/GYN at the University of Pennsylvania.

Although Macones and his collaborators didn't look at the hospitals' primary C-section rates—the proportion of patients without a prior cesarean who

In the Beginning . . .

A British traveler named R.W. Felkin described a successful cesarean delivery he'd observed in Uganda in 1879, and it sounds like the Ugandans' technique was more advanced than that of Westerners at the time. The Ugandan healer actually gave the woman banana wine to make her slightly drunk. At the time, most Westerners were performing the operation on unanesthetized women who needed to be held down by four or five men. In addition, the healer washed his hands with the stuff, which, because of its alcoholic content, must have killed at least some germs. Hand washing was a foreign concept to Western doctors at the time. Their credo: Grimy hands are busy, important hands.

The Ugandan woman's abdominal wound was pinned with iron needles and covered with a paste made from chewed roots. That might not sound very sanitary, but Felkin reported that the wound had entirely healed 11 days after the operation, and mom and baby were doing fine.

ended up having one—"I would bet that high primary section rates and low VBAC rates go hand-in-hand," Macones says. "It speaks to the tone of a hospital about the importance of the C-section rates. Some hospitals think it is important and really try to keep the [primary C-section] rate down, and others don't seem to be as interested in that."

Take South Miami Hospital and Baptist Hospital, sister institutions in Florida. South Miami doctors deliver about 3,500 babies every year; Baptist doctors, 4,000. Of all those births, fewer than a half-dozen at each hospital are successful VBACs, says Javier Vizoso, M.D., director of obstetrics and gynecology at South Miami and Baptist. "There are some doctors there who are just flat-out refusing to let women try," says Vizoso. That could help explain why South Miami's C-section rate—42 percent—led the state in 2001. Vizoso believes several factors are at work: "Part of it is [the doctors] feel it's not a safe thing to do; part of it is [the doctors] say, 'Listen, in today's environment, with the reimbursement the way it is, for me to sit in labor and delivery without moving is simply just too impractical.'" Clearly, if you want to attempt a VBAC in South Florida, you should avoid Vizoso's hospitals and the doctors who deliver there. No matter where you live, your best bet is to find a pro-VBAC doctor who delivers at a VBAC-friendly hospital.

TO TRY OR NOT TO TRY:
MOST VBAC ATTEMPTS ARE SUCCESSFUL

About 60 percent to 80 percent of women who try to deliver vaginally after a C-section do so. If you want to be one of them, find a doctor whose VBAC success rate is near the top of that range and whose overall C-section rate is lower than the average in your area. Even if you already attended childbirth education classes during a previous pregnancy, sign up for a refresher or, preferably, a course specifically designed for VBAC candidates.

Juliet, 33, was determined to have a VBAC. She delivered her first daughter by cesarean 3 years ago after 18 hours of labor and 2½ hours of pushing. The baby was "sunny-side up" instead of the usual face-down, making for a more difficult birth. Even though you could see the top of the baby's head, Juliet says, her doctor decided to perform a C-section. "I basically went through my entire labor. The only thing I didn't do was push the baby all the way out. I didn't have the satisfaction of completing it," she says now.

She'd come so close, she was certain she could deliver her next baby vaginally. But when she told her obstetrician she wanted to attempt a VBAC, he was less than agreeable. "There's a real high risk," he told her, relating one of the scarier stories he'd heard. Juliet was not dissuaded. "I was determined, because I had a really difficult recovery from the first C-section," she explains. "I had the typical 4 days in the hospital, but I felt really incapacitated. Now that I had a child at home, I didn't want to be in the hospital for 4 days. If there was no medical reason for me not to do a VBAC, I was going to do it."

Still, she worried a lot that her second labor and delivery would proceed much like her first: hours and hours of contractions,

TALKING POINT

Before settling on a doctor, ask what proportion of her patients who attempt a VBAC actually succeed. Look for a success rate of around 75 percent.

hours of pushing, all for naught. "I thought about it, but it still didn't make a difference to me. I guess I had nothing to lose. To me, it was really important to have the opportunity to try."

Juliet doesn't consider herself to be particularly confrontational, but the more she pressured her doctor, the more vehement he became. He asked her to sign a document waiving her right to sue if something unexpected happened to her or the baby when she tried for a VBAC. Finally, 33 weeks into her pregnancy, Juliet's doctor fired her. Get another doctor, he told her. "It totally shocked me when he said that. I don't think I was being that out of line," she says. Probably most patients and more than a few doctors would agree that she wasn't out of line—*he* was.

A friend was expecting around the same time as Juliet. Only her friend was certain she wanted another C-section, not a VBAC, and her doctor kept trying to talk her out of it. Juliet figured that was the doctor for her. After another lengthy labor and a lot of pushing, Juliet, who had added 50 pounds to her normal 105 while pregnant, delivered her 9 pound, 4 ounce baby. As Juliet discovered, you could save yourself a lot of aggravation by recognizing that it's virtually impossible to change a doctor's views about VBACs. But you can change doctors, and the earlier you do that, the better.

Words from the Wise

If you want to attempt a VBAC, sign up for a childbirth refresher course. Even better, sign up for a course aimed at VBAC candidates.

Like Juliet, Rashawna had a difficult recovery after delivering her firstborn, now age 8, by an emergency cesarean. His heart rate had kept dropping during labor, which led her doctor to recommend a C-section. Rashawna, who's now 28, didn't feel like her old self for more than 6 weeks after giving birth. That long abdominal incision really hurt. "I didn't want to go through that again for anything," she says.

So when she got pregnant a second time, one of the first things she asked her obstetrician was whether she had to have another C-section. Many people had told her she would. Not her doctor, though. "She said no, I had a choice," Rashawna recalls. "I could try a vaginal if I really wanted to." As with her first child, Rashawna's second baby was in no hurry to come out. Again, she went past her due date. Again, her doctor induced labor. After 8 hours of labor, Rashawna delivered her daughter, now age 3, vaginally. And even though she already had another child at home, it only took her about 2 weeks to recover from the vaginal delivery.

In Karen's case, her obstetrician was more eager for her to try a VBAC than she was. "I was on the fence," says Karen, 33, who delivered her first son, now age 1½, by emergency C-section because she was not fully dilated after 15 hours of labor. At her first birth, she was dilating fine until her cervix was 8½ centimeters—and then for 3 hours she made no further progress. At that point, Karen finally had to agree with her doctor that she needed to have a cesarean. "The recovery was so hard with the C-section," she recalls. "A day later I was still needing help to go to the potty." When it came time to plan for the second birth, she took into account the fact that her son would be only 16 months old when his younger sibling was born. If she had another cesarean, there was no way she'd be able to carry her first son upstairs to his crib every night.

Even so, up until a week before the birth of her second son, Karen still wasn't sure if she wanted to try to deliver vaginally. "It wasn't a decision to make lightly. My husband said, 'What if it doesn't work? I don't want to see you in that pain again. Why not just get up

at 6 o'clock in the morning and an hour later have the baby born?'"
But the doctor who had performed her cesarean was certain she
could do it. "Her confidence put me over," Karen says. "If she hadn't
done the surgery, then I wouldn't have the faith in her that I did."
That faith was not misplaced. Karen arrived at the hospital around
midnight and delivered her second son vaginally at 7:00 A.M.

A landmark new study suggests that your VBAC experience
is likely to be just as favorable. The study, sponsored by the National
Institute of Child Health and Human Development, is one of the
largest ever on the subject of VBACs. Researchers at 19 academic
medical centers joined forces to collect information about nearly
46,000 patients who'd previously had a C-section. The participa-
tion of so many institutions means the results are more likely to
apply to your own doctor and hospital than if they'd come from a
study at just a single hospital. A little more than a third of the
women, or about 16,000, scheduled repeat cesareans even though
there was no medical reason to prevent a VBAC. Nearly 40 percent, or about 18,000 attempted VBACs, and about three out of
four of them were successful. The remaining women had any of a
variety of medical reasons for not attempting a VBAC, such as severe preeclampsia or a suspected extra-large baby due to diabetes,
so they were excluded from the analysis.

While women who attempted VBACs did have a higher risk
of complications such as uterine rupture, the actual number of
problems was reassuringly small, says Ohio State's Landon, the
study's lead researcher. Out of the approximately 18,000 women
who tried VBACs, only 124 experienced a detectable uterine rupture. There were no uterine ruptures among the women who
scheduled repeat C-sections. Often, uterine tears are so small they
they can simply be stitched up or heal on their own. And even most
babies born to moms who have a much bigger uterine rupture do
just fine, Landon says.

Other differences between the study's VBAC and repeat C-section groups were equally small. For example, about 3 percent of the women who attempted a VBAC developed endometritis—an inflammation of the lining of the uterus—compared to about 2 percent of the elective repeat C-section group. Endometritis occurs when bacteria travel up from the vagina and into the uterus during labor. Most cases are cured with intravenous antibiotics followed by a course of oral antibiotics.

Words from the Wise

Although the thought of a uterine rupture might be enough to make you schedule a repeat C-section, remember that the majority of babies—not to mention their moms—whose mothers have such a tear do just fine.

While a preplanned cesarean generally is safer for moms and babies than one performed after hours of labor, it does have at least one drawback: Babies delivered by repeat elective cesareans are more likely to develop a respiratory condition called transient tachypnea of the newborn, or TTN, than babies whose moms labored, no matter how they ended up delivering. TTN is the main reason why newborns end up in the intensive care unit. A 1-year study of all mothers with a prior C-section who gave birth at Cleveland's Case Western Reserve University found that 6 percent of babies delivered by planned C-section developed TTN, compared to only 3 percent of babies delivered vaginally.

WEIGHT(Y) MATTERS: FACTORS THAT INFLUENCE YOUR CHANCES OF A SUCCESSFUL VBAC

Some OB/GYNs have taken up the challenge to figure out which women are the best candidates for a VBAC. That's important,

> ### Words from the Wise
>
> *If you're aiming for a VBAC, let labor begin and progress naturally, without the help of any drugs. If that is impossible, you and your baby should be monitored closely in a hospital capable of performing an emergency cesarean if necessary.*

because you'd rather not end up with a C-section after hours of labor. While researchers haven't yet come up with the equivalent of a crystal ball, they have identified certain factors that might increase your chances of having a successful VBAC.

You go into labor naturally. The University of Washington VBAC study mentioned earlier in this chapter found that women whose labor was induced with a type of drug called a prostaglandin were 15 times more likely to have a uterine rupture than women who had repeat C-sections without labor. While prostaglandins such as misoprostol (Cytotec) appear to be the most dangerous, inducing or revving up labor with Pitocin—the synthetic version of oxytocin—may also raise the risk of uterine rupture in women attempting a VBAC.

You've had only one C-section. If you want to try a VBAC, some studies suggest that it's best if you've had no more than one previous C-section. Of those who attempted VBACs in Landon's study, there were 11 uterine ruptures among the 984 women who had more than one prior C-section, for a rate of 1.12 percent. There were 114 uterine ruptures out of the 16,913 women who had only one prior C-section, for a rate of 0.67 percent. But the study didn't have enough women who'd had more than one C-section to be certain that they really did have nearly twice the risk of uterine rupture as those with only one prior cesarean. The difference between the two groups could have simply been due to chance.

Kathryn, 41, may hold some sort of C-section/VBAC record. Back in 1993, when the U.S. VBAC rate was still rising and malpractice awards weren't, she delivered her fourth child vaginally after three prior cesareans. Not only that, but she went on to deliver babies five, six and seven vaginally, too. By the time she conceived baby number eight, though, her doctor advised her that the chance of a rupture was high. "He wanted to do a planned section. I really fought it. I really didn't want to do that." She followed his advice, though. "That turned out to be my most beautiful delivery. With so many kids, it was nice to have it planned." She didn't stop there. Kathryn delivered her ninth child, now 16 months old, via planned cesarean as well. And, if you must know, she and her husband are open to having a 10th baby, too, although some doctors would say she'd be really pushing her luck after five C-sections, which may have raised her risk not only of a uterine rupture but of dangerous placenta abnormalities as well.

You've waited to get pregnant. You can help influence your luck with VBAC even before you try to conceive. For one, you want to avoid getting pregnant too soon after your cesarean. In a study of women who attempted VBACs, researchers at Boston's Brigham and Women's Hospital found that those who delivered more than 19 months after their C-section were two-thirds less likely to have a symptomatic uterine rupture. Their study included 2,409 women who delivered over a 12-year period. A second study at the University of California, Irvine, published a year later, focused on 1,185 women trying for a VBAC. Researchers found no difference in the uterine rupture rate based on how much time had elapsed between a cesarean and a VBAC attempt. However, among women who were induced, those giving birth more than 19 months after a cesarean were more likely to have a successful VBAC than those delivering 19 months or less after the C-section. In other words, your best bet is to wait at least 9 or 10 months after a C-section before trying to conceive again.

You conceive when you're close to your ideal weight. To ensure success with your VBAC, you need to watch your weight before conception as well as afterward. In a recent study, University of Mississippi OB/GYNs found that patients who weighed less than 200 pounds before getting pregnant had a VBAC success rate of 82 percent, compared to only 13 percent in patients who weighed more than 300 pounds. The success rate in women who weighed 200 pounds to 300 pounds was 57 percent.

Try not to gain too much weight during your pregnancy, or you could end up with a baby too big to fit through your pelvis. A recent study of women attempting VBACs at 16 community and university hospitals suggests that carrying a baby weighing more than 8.8 pounds can reduce the success rate in some women. Unfortunately, it's difficult to predict a baby's weight before birth, let alone whether mom's pelvis is big enough to deliver junior vaginally. Pelvimetry, or x-rays of the pelvis, have been shown to be pretty useless in predicting who's likely to have a successful vaginal delivery. But just because your first baby was too large to deliver vaginally doesn't mean that you won't be able to birth

Words from the Wise

If you've just delivered your first baby by C-section but hope to deliver your next baby vaginally, don't try to get pregnant right away. You'll lower your risk of a uterine rupture if your kids are born at least 19 months apart.

your next one vaginally.

Your prior deliveries were straightforward and uncomplicated. Clearly, two factors related to previous deliveries increase your chances of having a successful VBAC: Your C-section was performed for reasons unlikely to recur in subsequent pregnancies, such as a breech baby. And you've already had a vaginal delivery, either before or after your C-section. An-

Words from the Wise

You've already learned that being overweight when you conceive, or packing on too many pounds while pregnant can raise your risk of having a C-section. So it may not surprise you to learn that the same factors can also lower your chances of having a successful VBAC.

other study by researchers at Boston's Brigham and Women's Hospital suggests a third factor related to your prior cesarean: If you ran a fever above 100.4 degrees after your C-section, your risk of a uterine rupture in a trial of labor may be four times that of a woman who did not have a fever after her C-section. Scientists aren't yet sure how infection and poor wound healing, which cause fevers after a cesarean delivery, contribute to future risk of uterine rupture.

Your body and baby are cooperating. The American College of Obstetricians and Gynecologists lists a couple of other conditions that enhance your chances of a successful VBAC: a large enough pelvis and a baby who's head-down and unaccompanied. (A few small studies suggest that even if you're carrying twins, you might still be able to have a VBAC.)

Your prior incision was horizontal. A low horizontal, not a "classical," or high vertical, incision on the uterus also puts you in a good position. The lower part of the uterus is thinner and heals with a stronger scar than the upper part.

> ## Words from the Wise
>
> *Don't assume that the scar on your uterus runs in the same direction as the scar on your abdomen. Only your medical records can provide the answer. The reason this is important is because low horizontal uterine scars are less likely to tear during a trial of labor than high vertical scars.*

Anne, 44, found out the hard way that you can't judge your uterine scar by the one on your skin. Only your medical records know for sure. Anne became pretty sick from a wound infection after delivering her first son, now 19, by cesarean. He was breech. Anne was looking forward to delivering her second son, now 16, by VBAC. Halfway through that pregnancy, though, Anne's doctor informed her that she had a vertical scar on her uterus, even though the one on her belly was horizontal. "I was just flabbergasted, and I was so angry when I found out that I had to have a C-section again," she recalls. Two years later, she delivered her third son by cesarean.

You're on the younger side. Some research suggests that younger women might have an edge over older women when it comes to VBACs. A review of the medical records of all women who attempted a VBAC during a 12-year period at Boston's Brigham and Women's Hospital found that women 30 and older were three times more likely to experience a uterine rupture than younger women. Even for women 30 and older, though, the risk was only 3 percent, compared to 1 percent for the younger women. Patients in their 40s did have an even higher rate of uterine rupture, but there weren't enough women in that age group to determine whether the increased risk was real or merely due to chance. The researchers acknowledge that they can't be sure that the 30- and 40-something women's age is what boosted their rupture risk. There might have been other, unidentified factors more common in older women (rather than just their age) that increased their rupture risk.

TO EACH HER OWN: SCHEDULING A REPEAT C-SECTION

Maybe your pregnancy history suggests that you're not a good candidate for a VBAC. Or perhaps you'd just rather not gamble on attempting one. You're concerned about the uterine rupture risk, no matter how low it is, and you're not enamored of the possibility of going through labor and ending up with an unplanned C-section. Perhaps you can identify with women who ask to deliver their first baby by cesarean because they like the idea of being able to schedule their baby's birth. You have one advantage over them: Unlike women who've never had a C-section, you have a pretty clear idea of what you're getting into when you schedule one.

Casey's first daughter, now age 3½, needed to be delivered by emergency cesarean 10 weeks before her due date. When Casey got pregnant again 3 years later, her doctor told her she had a 60 percent chance of delivering the baby vaginally. But, Casey says now, "I just preferred not going through labor and then ending up having to have a C-section." So, in her 34th week, she scheduled a cesarean. Casey's friends were surprised. "They knew when I had my first C-section how hard my recovery was. They asked me: Are you sure you want to go through that again? They tried to convince me otherwise, but it didn't work," Casey says. "Sometimes I think you forget the pain."

Having a preplanned C-section just made it easier as far as her family and job were concerned, says Casey, 27, a rural letter carrier. "Everybody took off work. It wasn't this rush thing. We were all at the hospital at 7:00 A.M." And she was able to tell her supervisor at the post office the exact date she'd be back at work. "I don't have regrets at all about having a C-section. It hurt, but if I had another kid, I'd probably do it again."

Thirty-four-year-old Lisa can relate. Her son, who's now 3, was breech. She ended up delivering him by cesarean after a failed version attempt. She's only a third of the way through her second pregnancy, but she's already pretty sure she knows how she wants to deliver. Although it's unlikely that her second baby will also be breech, "I think I'm going to have a scheduled C-section, because I feel like I know what to expect," she says. "If I can plan and work things through and have a general idea of what's going to happen, I can do okay."

Like Lisa, Sue, 36, felt comfortable delivering her second daughter, now 3 months old, via repeat C-section because that's the only way she knew. The final straw was that her trusted doctor advised against attempting a VBAC because of the rupture risk. Sue's sister-in-law had a C-section with her third child and then had a VBAC with her fourth. "I just didn't have any aspirations about going through labor and delivering that way," says Sue. "My mother-in-law said, 'Don't think you missed out on anything.'" Sue delivered her firstborn, now age 2, by emergency cesarean more than 5 weeks early because she developed an unusual condition that greatly raised her blood pressure. A friend had to drive her to the hospital because her lawyer husband was in a trial. That's another reason a planned repeat C-section was so appealing. "I just thought it would be really cool to schedule when you're going to have your child and actually have it on that day," she says. Her doctor wanted to perform the surgery 2 weeks before her due date, but Sue objected because husband was going to be in another trial then. The C-section was set for a week before her due date. This time, Sue's husband was going to get to drive her to the hospital.

Beth, 36, delivered her first child vaginally, but she had an emergency cesarean with her second, because her labor wasn't progressing and his heart rate kept dropping. She's now 2½ months pregnant with her third child, and she's already informed her obstetrician that she wants another C-section. "I liked it so much better" than her vaginal delivery, she says. "I had such a great C-section experience, I don't know why I wouldn't do it again." With the birth of her first child, now 6, "I just felt I had been beaten up. It took me a lot longer to feel like I could walk around and function normally." With the C-section, "I felt it was like a much more controlled healing process."

Memories of painful contractions from an unmedicated and unsuccessful labor drove Gigi, 42, to swear off any attempts at a VBAC. Her firstborn, now 18, was delivered by emergency cesarean. "Five years later, when I became pregnant again, I was dismayed to have a doctor who acted virtuous about VBACs. She told me that a VBAC was better for me, as there was less of a risk of adhesions, and it would be better for the baby. I considered her argument for about 2 seconds. It didn't take me long to recall what I'd gone through before," she says now.

After she rejected the idea of trying for a VBAC, Gigi says, she never could

Words from the Wise

Don't beat yourself up or let anyone make you feel guilty about scheduling a repeat cesarean instead of attempting a VBAC. You should make the choice that's best for you. Some women feel more comfortable going with another C-section because they already know what to expect.

get another appointment with that doctor. "One of the other doctors in the practice would see me. The senior physician in the practice told me that he thought I had made the best choice," she said. He told Gigi, "I'm doing a VBAC later this morning, and, frankly, it scares the hell out of me." Gigi went on to deliver children three and four, now ages 7 and 6, by elective cesarean as well. With so many C-sections, though, she's lucky she never had her uterus rupture or had her placenta develop abnormally.

Your notion of an ideal delivery might be more like Juliet's than Gigi's, or it might not. As this book has repeatedly pointed out, one-size-fits-all applies to receiving blankets, not childbirth. No one can guarantee that your delivery will go exactly as you'd like, but you can improve the odds by learning about your options and picking a doctor or midwife who shares your philosophy. And remember—your mode of delivery has nothing to do with your worth as a mother. Enjoy your new baby!

BIBLIOGRAPHY

CHAPTER 1

Alarab M, Regan C, O'Connell MP, Keane DP, O'Herlihy C, Foley ME. Singleton vaginal breech delivery at term: still a safe option. *Obstetrics & Gynecology* 2004; 103:407-412.

American College of Obstetricians and Gynecologists Committee Opinion. Mode of Term Singleton Breech Delivery. No. 265; December 2001.

American College of Obstetricians and Gynecologists Practice Bulletin. External cephalic version. No. 13; February 2000.

American College of Obstetricians and Gynecologists Committee Opinion. Placenta accreta. No. 266; January 2002.

American College of Obstetricians and Gynecologists Practice Bulletin. Management of herpes in pregnancy. No. 8; October 1999.

American College of Obstetricians and Gynecologists Practice Bulletin. Shoulder dystocia. No. 40; November 2002.

Bernstein, Sharon. County C-section rule took heavy human toll. *Los Angeles Times,* January 25, 1998.

Blickstein I, Goldman RD, Kupfermine M. Delivery of breech first twins: a multicenter retrospective study. *Obstetrics & Gynecology* 2000; 95:37-42.

Brown ZA, Wald A, Morrow RA, Selke S, Zeh J, Corey L. Effect of seriologic status and cesarean delivery on transmission rates of herpes simplex virus from mother to infant. *Journal of the American Medical Association* 2003; 289:203-209.

Callaghan WM, Berg CJ. Pregnancy-related mortality among women aged 35 years and older, United States, 1991-1997. *Obstetrics & Gynecology* 2003; 102:1015-1021.

Cardini F, Weixin H. Moxibustion for correction of breech presentation: a randomized controlled trial. *Journal of the American Medical Association* 1998; 280:1580-1584.

Cohan D. Cesarean delivery and risk of herpes simplex virus infection. *Journal of the American Medical Association* 2003; 289:2208.

Daniel I, Berg C, Johnson CH, Atrash H. Magnitude of maternal morbidity during labor and delivery: United States 1993-1997. *American Journal of Public Health* 2003; 93:631-634.

Dominguez KL, Lindegren M, D'Almada PJ et al. Increasing trend of cesarean deliveries in HIV-infected women in the United States from 1994-2000. *Journal of the Acquired Immune Deficiency Syndrome* 2003; 333:232-238.

Fitzpatrick M, McQuillan K, O'Herlihy C. Influence of persistent occiput posterior position on delivery outcome. *Obstetrics & Gynecology* 2001; 98:1027-1031.

Gabert HA, Bey M. History and development of cesarean operation. *Obstetrics and Gynecology Clinics of North America* 1988; 15:591-605.

Gerrero S, Bentivoglio G. Post-operative complications after caesarean section in HIV-infected women. *Archives of Gynecology and Obstetrics* 2003; 268:268-73.

Gifford, DS, Morton SC, Fiske M, Keesey J, Keeler E, Kahn KI. Lack of progress in labor as a reason for cesarean. *Obstetrics & Gynecology* 2000; 95:589-595

Gilbert WM, Hicks SM, Boe NM, Danielsen B. Vaginal versus cesarean delivery for breech presentation in California: a population-based study. *Obstetrics & Gynecology* 2003; 102:911-917.

Gregory KD, Korst LM, Krychman M, Cane P, Platt LD. Variation in vaginal breech delivery rates by hospital type. *Obstetrics & Gynecology* 2001; 97:385-390.

Hannah ME, Hannah WJ, Hewson SA, Hodnett ED, Saigal S, Willan AR. Planned caesarean section versus planned vaginal birth for breech presentation at term: a randomised multicentre trial. Term Breech Trial Collaborative Group. *Lancet* 2000; 356:1375-1383.

Hannah ME, Hannah WJ, Hodnett ED, Chalmers B, Kung R et al. Outcomes at 3 months after planned cesarean vs. planned vaginal delivery for breech presentation at term. *Journal of the American Medical Association* 2002; 287:1822-1831.

Heffner LJ, Elkin E, Fretts RC. Impact of labor induction, gestational age, and maternal age on cesarean delivery rates. *Obstetrics & Gynecology* 2003; 102:287-293.

Hofmeyr G. Interventions to help external cephalic version for breech presentation at term. *Cochrane Database of Systematic Reviews* 2004; (1):CD000184.

Hofmeyr GJ, Hannah ME. Planned caesarean section for term breech delivery. *Cochrane Database of Systematic Reviews*. 2003 (3); CD000166.

Hofmeyr GJ, Kulier R. Hands/knees posture in late pregnancy or labour for fetal malposition (lateral or posterior). *The Cochrane Database of Systematic Reviews* (Complete Reviews) 2004, (1). DOI: 10.1002/14651858.CD001063.

Hogle KL, Hutton EK, McBrien KA, Barrett JER, Hannah ME. Cesarean delivery for twins: a systematic review and meta-analysis. *American Journal of Obstetrics and Gynecology* 2003; 188:220-227.

Hutton EK, Kaufman K, Hodnett E, Amankwah K, Hewson SA, McKay D, Szalai JP, Hannah ME. External cephalic version beginning at 34 weeks' gestation versus 37 weeks' gestation: a randomized multicenter trial. *American Journal of Obstetrics & Gynecology* 2003; 189:245-254.

Jolly MC, Sebire NJ, Harris JP, Regan L, Robinson S. Risk factors for macrosomia and its clinical consequences: a study of 350,311 pregnancies. *European Journal of Obstetrics & Gynecology and Reproductive Biology* 2003; 111:9-14.

Kariminia A, Chamberlain ME, Keogh J, Shea A. Randomised controlled trial of effect of hands and knees posturing on incidence of occiput posterior position at birth., *BMJ* 2004 Feb 28; 328(7438):490. Epub 2004 Jan 26.

Krebs L, Langhoff-Roos J. Elective cesarean delivery for term breech. *Obstetrics & Gynecology* 2003; 101:690-696.

Leeman L, Leeman R. A Native American community with a 7% cesarean delivery rate: Does case mix, ethnicity, or labor management explain the low rate? *Annals of Family Medicine* 2003; 1:36-43.

Lieberman E, Cohen A, Lang J, Frigoletto F, Goetzl L. Maternal intrapartum temperature elevation as a risk factor for cesarean delivery and assisted vaginal delivery. *American Journal of Public Health* 1999; 89:506-510.

Longo SA, Dola CP, Pridjian G. Preeclampsia and eclampsia revisited. *Southern Medical Journal* 2003; 96:891-899.

Martin JA, Hamilton BE, Sutton PD, Ventura SJ, Menacker F, Munson ML. Births: final data for 2002. *National Vital Statistics Reports* 2003; Vol. 52, No. 10.

Mattar F, Sibai BM. Prevention of preeclampsia. *Seminars in Perinatology* 1999; 23:58-64.

Mostello D, Droll DA, Bierig SM, Cruz-Flores S, Leet T. Tertiary care improves the chance for vaginal delivery in women with preeclampsia. *American Journal of Obstetrics and Gynecology* 2003; 189:824-829.

Nassar AH, Usta IM, Rechdan JB, Harb TS, Adra AM, Abu-Musa AA. Pregnancy outcome in spontaneous twins versus twins who were conceived through in vitro fertilization. *American Journal of Obstetrics and Gynecology* 2003; 189:513-518.

Pattinson RC. Pelvimetry for fetal cephalic presentations at term. *Cochrane Database of Systematic Reviews* 2000;(2):CD000161.

Ponkey SE. Cohen AP, Heffner LJ, Lieberman E. Persistent fetal occiput posterior position: obstetric outcomes. *Obstetrics & Gynecology* 2003; 101:915-920.

Pressman EK, Bienstock JL, Blakemore KJ, Martin SA, Callan NA. Prediction of birth weight by ultrasound in the third trimester. *Obstetrics & Gynecology* 2000; 95:502-506.

Queenan JT. Teaching infrequently used skills: vaginal breech delivery. *Obstetrics & Gynecology* 2004; 103:405-406.

Remsberg KE, McFarland KF, McKeown RE, Irwin LS. Diabetes in pregnancy and cesarean delivery. *Diabetes Care* 1999; 22:1561-1567.

Rucker MP, Rucker EM. A librarian looks at cesarean section. *Bulletin of the History of Medicine* 1951; 25:132-148.

Schwartz R, Teramo KA. What is the significance of macrosomia? *Diabetes Care* 1999; 22:1201-1205.

Sewell JE. Cesarean section—a brief history. *American College of Obstetricians and Gynecologists*; 1993.

Sheffield JS, Hollier LM, Hill JB, Stuart GS, Wendel GD. Acyclovir prophylaxis to prevent herpes simplex virus recurrence at delivery: a systematic review. *Obstetrics & Gynecology* 2003; 102:1396-1403.

Sibony O, Touitou S, Luton D, Oury JF, Blot PH. A comparison of the neonatal morbidity of second twins to that of a low-risk population. *European Journal of Obstetrics & Gynecology and Reproductive Biology* 2003; 108:157-163.

Trolle F. The History of Caesarean Section. C.A. Reitzel Booksellers, Copenhagen: 1982.

Varner MW, Fraser AM, Hunter CY, Corneli PS, Ward RH. The intergenerational predisposition to operative delivery. *Obstetrics & Gynecology* 1996; 87:905-911.

Weber CS. Postmortem cesarean section: review of the literature and case reports. *American Journal of Obstetrics and Gynecology* 1971; 110:158-165.

Weeks JW, Pitman T, Spinnato JA 2nd. Fetal macrosomia: Does antenatal prediction affect delivery route and birth outcome? *American Journal of Obstetrics and Gynecology* 1995; 173:1215-1219.

Wen SW, Fung KFK, Oppenheimer L, Demissie K, Yang Q, Walker M. Occurrence and predictors of cesarean delivery for the second twin after vaginal delivery of the first twin. *Obstetrics & Gynecology* 2004; 103:413-419.

Wilkes PT, Wolf DM, Kronbach DW, Kunze M, Gibbs RS. Risk factors for cesarean delivery at presentation of nulliparous patients in labor. *Obstetrics & Gynecology* 2003; 102:1352-1357.

Williams KP, Galerneau F. Intrapartum influences on cesarean delivery in multiple gestation. *Acta Obstetrica et Gynecologica Scandinavica* 2003; 82:241-245.

Zhang J, Troendle JF, Yancey MK. Reassessing the labor curve in nulliparous women women. *American Journal of Obstetrics and Gynecology* 2002; 187:824-828.

CHAPTER 2

American College of Obstetricians and Gynecologists Patient Information Pamphlet. *Cesarean Birth.* March 1999.

American College of Surgeons. About cesarean childbirth. http://www.facs.org/public_info/operation/cesarean.pdf

Boley JP. The history of caesarean section. *Canadian Medical Association Journal* 1991; 145:319-322.

Dewey KG, Monnsen-Rivers LA, Heinig MJ, Cohen RJ. Risk factors for suboptimal infant breastfeeding behavior, delayed onset of lactation, and excess neonatal weight loss. *Pediatrics* 2003; 112:607-619.

Hem E, Bordahl PE. Max Sanger. Father of the modern caesarean section. *Gynecologic and Obstetric Investigation* 2003; 55:127-129.

Jakobi P, Solt I, Tamir A, Zimmer EZ. Over-the-counter oral analgesia for postcesarean pain. *American Journal of Obstetrics and Gynecology* 2002; 187:1066-1069.

Mangesi L, Hofmeyr GJ. Early compared with delayed oral fluids and food after caesarean section. *Cochrane Database of Systematic Reviews* 2002; (3):CD0035.

March of Dimes. *C-section.* www.marchofdimes.com/pnhec/240_1031.asp.

Normand MC, Damato EG. Postcesarean infection. *Journal of Obstetric, Gynecologic, and Neonatal Nursing* 2001; 30:642-648.

Patolia DS, Hilliard RI, Toy EC, Baker B. Early feeding after cesarean: randomized trial. *Obstetrics & Gynecology* 2001 Jul;98:113-6.

Smaill F, Hofmeyr GJ. Antibiotic prophylaxis for cesarean section. *Cochrane Database of Systematic Reviews* 2002; (3):CD000933.

Trolle F. *The History of Caesarean Section.* C.A. Reitzel Booksellers, Copenhagen: 1982.

CHAPTER 3

American College of Obstetricians and Gynecologists Patient Information Pamphlet. *Cesarean Birth.* March 1999.

American College of Surgeons. *About cesarean childbirth.* http://www.facs.org/public_info/operation/cesarean.pdf

Baumann LS, Spencer J. The effects of topical vitamin E on the cosmetic appearance of scars. *Dermatological Surgery* 1999; 24:311-315.

Declercq ER, Sakala C, Corry MP, Applebaum S, Risher P. *Listening to Mothers: Report of the First National U.S. Survey of Women's Childbearing Experiences.* New York: Maternity Center Association, October 2002.

March of Dimes. *C-section.* www.marchofdimes.com/pnhec/240_1031.asp.

CHAPTER 4

Allen VM, O'Connell CM, Liston RM, Baskett TF. Maternal morbidity associated with cesarean delivery without labor compared with spontaneous onset of labor at term. *Obstetrics & Gynecology* 2003; 102:1-6.

Almeida EC, Nogueira AA, Candido dos Reis FJ, Rosa e Silva JC. Cesarean section as a cause of chronic pelvic pain. *International Journal of Gynaecology and Obstetrics* 2002; 79:101-104.

American College of Obstetricians and Gynecologists Committee Opinion. *Surgery and patient choice: the ethics of decision making.* No. 289; November 2003.

American College of Obstetricians and Gynecologists Committee Opinion. *Placenta accreta.* No. 266: January 2002.

American College of Obstetricians and Gynecologists. Task Force on Cesarean Delivery Rates. *Evaluation of cesarean delivery;* 2000.

Boley JP. The history of caesarean section. *Canadian Medical Association Journal* 1991; 145:319-322.

Buchsbaum GM, Chin M, Glantz C, Guzick D. Prevalence of urinary incontinence and associated risk factors in a cohort of nuns. *Obstetrics & Gynecology* 2002; 100:226-229.

Burgio KL, Zyczynski H, Locher JL, Richter HE, Redden DT, Wright KC. Urinary incontinence in the 12-month postpartum period. *Obstetrics & Gynecology* 2003; 102:1291-1298.

Clark SL, Hankins GD. Temporal and demographic trends in cerebral palsy-fact and fiction. *American Journal of Obstetrics and Gynecology* 2003; 188:628-633.

Davila GW. Urogynecologists are not encouraging a higher cesarean section rate. *American Journal of Obstetrics and Gynecology* 2003; 188:1660.

Davila GW. Informed consent for obstetrics management: a urogynecologic perspective. *International Urogynecology Journal and Pelvic Floor Dysfunction* 2001; 12:289-291.

Dietz HP, Bennett MJ. The effect of childbirth on pelvic organ mobility. *Obstetrics & Gynecology* 2003; 102:223-228.

Eckler R. Labour for two days? Uh, no thanks. *National Post;* Oct. 21, 2003.

Eggesbo M, Botten , Stigum H, Nafstad P, Magnus P. Is delivery by cesarean section a risk factor for food allergy? *Journal of Allergy and Clinical Immunology* 2003; 112:420-426.

Farrell SA, Allen VM, Baskett TF. Parturition and urinary incontinence in primiparas. *Obstetrics & Gynecology* 2001; 97:350-356.

Goldberg RP, Kwon C, Gandhi S, Atkuru LV, Sorensen M, Sand PK. Urinary incontinence among mothers of multiples: the protective effect of cesarean delivery. *American Journal of Obstetrics and Gynecology* 2003; 188:1447-1453.

Gould JB, Qin C, Marks AR, Chavez G. Neonatal mortality in weekend vs. weekday births. *Journal of the American Medical Association* 2003; 289:2958-2962.

Haas DM, Ayres AW. Laceration injury at cesarean section. *Journal of Maternal-Fetal & Neonatal Medicine* 2002; 11:196-198.

Hall C. Why should I have to go through the pain of childbirth? *The Daily Telegraph,* November 13, 2003.

Harer WB. Patient choice cesarean. *ACOG Clinical Review* 2000; 5;1,13,15-16.

Harper MA, Byington RP, Espeland MA, Naughton M, Meyer R, Lane K. Pregnancy-related death and health care services. *Obstetrics & Gynecology* 2003; 102:273-278.

Kacmar J, Bhimani L, Boyd M, Shah-Hosseini R, Peipert J. Route of delivery as a risk factor for emergent peripartum hysterectomy: a case-control study. *Obstetrics & Gynecology* 2003; 102:141-145.

Levine EM, Ghai V, Barton JJ, Strom CM. Mode of delivery and risk of respiratory diseases in newborns. *Obstetrics & Gynecology* 2001; 97:439-442.

Li T, Rhoads GG, Smulian J, Demissie K, Warternberg D, Kruse L. Physician cesarean delivery rates and risk-adjusted perinatal outcomes. *Obstetrics & Gynecology* 2003; 101:1204-1212.

Lydon-Rochelle M, Holt VL, Easterling TR, Martin DP. Cesarean delivery and postpartum mortality among primiparas in Washington State, 1987-1996. *Obstetrics & Gynecology*; 97:169-174.

Lydon-Rochelle M, Holt VL, Easterling TR, Martin DP. First-birth cesarean and placental abruption or previa at second birth(1). *Obstetrics & Gynecology* 2001; 97:765-769.

Lydon-Rochelle M, Holt VL, Martin DP. Delivery method and self-reported postpartum general health status among primiparous women. *Paediatric and Perinatal Epidemiology* 2001; 15:232-240.

Lydon-Rochelle M, Holt VL, Martin DP, Easterling TR. Association between method of delivery and maternal rehospitalization. *Journal of the American Medical Association* 2000; 283:2411-2416.

Maternity Center Association. *Listening to mothers: report of the first national U.S. survey of women's childbearing experiences.* New York: Maternity Center Association, October 2002.

Minkoff H, Chervenak FA. Elective primary cesarean delivery. *New England Journal of Medicine* 2003; 348:946-949.

National Center for Clinical Excellence. *Caesarean section clinical guideline.* April 2004, www.nice.org.uk

Nygaard I, Cruikshank DP. Should all women be offered elective cesarean delivery? *Obstetrics & Gynecology* 2003; 102:217-219.

Porter M, Bhattacharya S, van Teijlingen E, Templeton A. Does caesarean section cause infertility? *Human Reproduction* 2003; 18:1983-1986.

Quadros LGA. Brazilian obstetricians are pressured to perform caesarean sections. *BMJ* 2000; 320:1073.

Robson S, Ellwood D. Should obstetricians support a 'term cephalic trial'? *Australian and New Zealand Journal of Obstetrics and Gynaecology* 2003; 43:341-343.

Rortveit G, Daltveit AK, Hannestad YS, Hunskaar S. Urinary incontinence after vaginal delivery or cesarean section. *New England Journal of Medicine* 2003; 348:900-907.

Saisto T, Halmesmaki E. Fear of childbirth: a neglected dilemma. *Acta Obstetrica et Gynecologica Scandinavica* 2003; 82:201-208.

Schindl M, Birner P, Reingrabner M, Joura E, Husslein P, Langer M. Elective cesarean section vs. spontaneous delivery: a comparative study of birth experience. *Acta Obstetrica et Gynecologica Scandinavica* 2003; 82:834-840.

Smith GCS, Pell JP, Cameron AD, Dobbie R. Risk of perinatal death associated with labor after cesarean delivery in uncomplicated term pregnancies. *Journal of the American Medical Association* 2002; 287:2684-2690.

Smith GC, Wood AM, White IR, Pell JP, Cameron AD, Dobbie, R. Cesarean delivery and the risk of hospital admission for respiratory disease in childhood. Society for Gynecologic Investigation 2003 annual meeting; abstract 655.

Snowbeck C. More women are having babies without going through labor. But is it a good idea. *Pittsburgh Post-Gazette;* March 18, 2003.

Stephansson O, Dickman PW, Johansson AL, Kieler H, Cnattingius S. Time of birth and risk of intrapartum and early neonatal death. *Epidemiology* 2003; 14:218-222.

Sze EHM, Sherard GB, Dolezal JM. Pregnancy, labor, delivery, and pelvic organi prolapse. *Obstetrics & Gynecology* 2002; 100:981-986.

Towner D, Castro MA, Eby-Wilkens E, Gilbert WM. Effect of mode of delivery in nulliparous women on neonatal intracranial injury. *New England Journal of Medicine* 1999; 341:1709-1714.

Xu B, Pekkanen J, Hartikainen AL, Jarvelin MR. Caesarean section and risk of asthma and allergy in adulthood. *Journal of Allergy and Clinical Immunology* 2001; 107:732-733.

CHAPTER 5

Alexander JM, et al. Epidural analgesia lengthens the Friedman active phase of labor. *Obstetrics & Gynecology* 2002; 100:46-50.

American College of Obstetricians and Gynecologists Committee Opinion. Analgesia and cesarean delivery rates. No. 269; Feb. 2002.

American College of Obstetricians and Gynecologists. Task Force on Cesarean Delivery Rates. Evaluation of cesarean delivery; 2000.

Baeten JM, Bukuski EA, Lambe M. Pregnancy complications and outcomes among overweight and obese nulliparous women. *American Journal of Public Health* 2001; 91:436-440.

Crane SS, Wojtowycz MA, Dye TD, Aubry RH, Artal R. Association between pre-pregnancy obesity and the risk of cesarean delivery. *Obstetrics & Gynecology* 1997; 89:213-216.

Garcia F, Miller HB, Huggins GR, Gordon TA. Effect of academic affiliation and obstetric volume on clinical outcome and cost of childbirth. *Obstetrics & Gynecology* 2001; 97:567-576.

Gregory KD, Korst LM, Krychman MB, Cane P, Platt LD. Variation in vaginal breech delivery rates by hospital type. *Obstetrics & Gynecology* 2001; 97:385-390.

Halpern SH, Leighton BL, Ohlsson A, Barrett J, Rice A. Effect of epidural vs. parenteral opioid analgesia on the progress of labor. *Journal of the American Medical Association* 1998; 280:2105-2110.

Heffner LJ, Elkin E, Fretts RC. Impact of labor induction, gestational age, and maternal age on cesarean delivery rates. *Obstetrics & Gynecology* 2003; 102:287-293.

Hodnett ED. Caregiver support for women during childbirth. *Cochrane Database of Systematic Reviews* 2002; (1):CD000199.

Hodnett ED, et al. Effectiveness of nurses as providers of birth labor support in North American hospitals. *Journal of the American Medical Association* 2002; 288:1373-1381.

Jackson DJ, Lang JM, Swartz WH, Ganiats TG, Fullerton J, Ecker J, Nguyen U. Outcomes, safety, and resource utilization in a collaborative care birth center program compared with traditional physician-based perinatal care. *American Journal of Public Health* 2003; 93:999-1006.

Jensen DM, Damm P, Sorensen B, Molsted-Pedersen L, Westergaard JG, Ovesen P, Beck-Nielsen H. Pregnancy outcome and prepregnancy body mass index in 2459 glucose-tolerant Danish women. *American Journal of Obstetrics and Gynecology* 2003; 189:239-244.

Johnson DP, Davis NR, Brown AJ. Risk of cesarean delivery after induction at term in nulliparous women with an unfavorable cervix. *American Journal of Obstetrics and Gynecology* 2003; 188:1565-1569.

Joseph KS, Young DC, Dodds L, O'Connell CM, Allen VM, Chandra S, Allen AC. Changes in maternal characteristics and obstetric practice and recent increases in primary cesarean delivery. *Obstetrics & Gynecology* 2003; 102:791-800.

Lieberman E, Cohen A, Lang J, Frigoletto F, Goetzl L. Maternal intrapartum termperature elevation as a risk factor for cesarean delivery and assisted vaginal delivery. *American Journal of Public Health* 1999; 89:506-510.

MacDorman MF, Mathews TJ, Martin JA, Malloy MH. Trends and characteristics of induced labour in the United States, 1989-1998. *Paediatric and Perinatal Epidemiology* 2002; 16:263-273.

Mattingly J, D'Alessio J, Ramanathan J. Effects of obstetric analgesics and anesthetics on the neonate: a review. *Paediatric Drugs* 2003; 5:615-627.

Miller JM. First successful cesarean section in the British empire. *American Journal of Obstetrics and Gynecology* 1992; 166:269.

Murphy DJ, Pope C, Frost J, Liebling RE. Women's views on the impact of operative delivery in the second stage of labour: qualitative interview study. *BMJ* 2003; 327:1132-1135.

Myles TD, Gooch J, Santolaya J. Obesity as an independent risk factor for infectious morbidity in patients who undergo cesarean delivery. *Obstetrics & Gynecology* 2002;100:959-964.

Nuthalapaty FS, Rouse DJ, Owen J. The association of maternal weight with cesarean risk, labor duration, and cervical dilation rate during labor induction. *Obstetrics & Gynecology* 2004; 103:452-456.

Rayburn WF, Zhang J. Rising rates of labor induction: present concerns and future strategies. *Obstetrics & Gynecology* 2002; 100:164-167.

Rhodes JC, Schoendorf KC, Parker JD. Contribution of excess weight gain during pregnancy and macrosomia to the cesarean delivery rate, 1990-2000. *Pediatrics* 2003; 111:1181-1185.

Sanchez-Ramos L, Olivier F, Delke I, Kaunitz AM. Labor induction versus expectant management for postterm pregnancies: A systematic review with meta-analysis. *Obstetrics & Gynecology* 2003; 101:1312-1318.

Sheiner E, Levy A, Katz M, Mazor M. Short stature-an independent risk factor for cesarean delivery. Society for Maternal-Fetal Medicine annual meeting. February 2004.

Shepard MJ, Saftlas AF, Leo-Summers L, Bracken MB. Maternal anthropometric factors and risk of primary cesarean delivery. *American Journal of Public Health* 1998; 88:1534-1538.

Simpson KR, Atterbury J. Trends and issues in labor induction in the United States: implications for clinical practice. *Journal of Obstetrics, Gynocologic, and Neonatal Nursing* 2003; 32:767-779.

Stuart K, Krakauer H, Schone E, Lin M, Cheng E, Meyer GS. Labor epidurals improve outcomes for babies of mothers at high risk for unscheduled cesarean section. *Journal of Perinatology* 2001; 21:178-185.

Thacker SB, Stroup D, Chang M. Continuous electronic heart rate monitoring for fetal assessment during labor. *Cochrane Database of Systematic Reviews* 2001; (2):CD000063.

Towner D, Castro MA, Eby-Wilkens E, Gilbert WM. Effect of mode of delivery in nulliparous women on neonatal intracranial injury. *New England Journal of Medicine* 1999; 341:1709-1714.

Vahratian A, Zhang J, Troendle J, Siega-Riz AM, Savitz D, Thorp Jr. J. "Maternal obesity and labor progression in nulliparous women." Society for Maternal-Fetal Medicine annual meeting. February 2004.

Wood SH. Should women be given a choice about fetal assessment in labor? *MCN: The American Journal of Maternal/Child Nursing* 2003; 28:292-298.

Zhang J, Klebanoff MA, DerSimonian R. Epidural analgesia in association with duration of labor and mode of delivery: a quantitative review. *American Journal of Obstetrics and Gynecology* 1999; 180:970-977.

Zhang J, Troendle J, Vahratian A, Sciscione A, Hoffman M. "Elective labor induction and labor progression in nulliparas." Society for Maternal-Fetal Medicine annual meeting. February 2004.

Zhang J, Troendle JF, Yancey MK. Reassessing the labor curve in nulliparous women. *American Journal of Obstetrics and Gynecology* 2002; 187:824-828.

CHAPTER 6

American College of Obstetricians and Gynecologists Committee Opinion. "Induction of labor for vaginal birth after cesarean delivery." No. 271. April 2002.

American College of Obstetricians and Gynecologists Practice Bulletin. Vaginal birth after previous cesarean delivery. No. 5. July 1999.

Carr CA, Burkhardt P, Avery M. Vaginal birth after cesarean birth: a national survey of U.S. midwifery practice. *Journal of Midwifery and Women's Health* 2002; 47:347-52.

Carroll CS Sr, Magann EF, Chauhan SP, Klauser CK, Morrison JC. Vaginal birth after cesarean section versus elective repeat cesarean delivery: weight-based outcomes. *American Journal of Obstetrics and Gynecology* 2003; 188:1516-1520.

Chauhan SP, Magann EF, Wiggs CD, Barrilleaux PS, Martin JN Jr. Pregnancy after classic cesarean delivery. *Obstetrics & Gynecology* 2002; 100:946-950.

Cragin EB. Conservatism in obstetrics. *New York Medical Journal* 1916; 104:1-3.

Dinsmoor MJ, Brock EL. Predicting failed trial of labor after primary cesarean delivery. *Obstetrics & Gynecology* 2004; 103:282-286.

Dunsmoor-Su R, Sammel M, Stevens E, Peipert JL, Macones G. Impact of sociodemographic and hospital factors on attempts at vaginal birth after cesarean delivery. *Obstetrics & Gynecology* 2003; 102:1358-1365.

Fisler RE, Cohen A, Ringer SA, Lieberman E. Neonatal outcome after trial of labor compared with elective repeat cesarean section. *Birth* 2003; 30:83-88.

Flamm BL. Vaginal birth after caesarean (VBAC). Best Practice & Research. *Clinical Obstetrics & Gynaecology* 2001; 15:81-92.

Flamm BL. Vaginal birth after cesarean: What's new in the new millennium? *Current Opinions in Obstetrics and Gynecology* 2002; 14:595-9.

Greene MF. Vaginal delivery after cesarean section - is the risk acceptable? *New England Journal of Medicine* 2001; 345:54-55.

Gregory KD, Korst LM, Cane P, Platt LD, Kahn K. Vaginal birth after cesarean and uterine rupture rates in California. *Obstetrics & Gynecology*; 94:985-989.

Gregory KD, Korst LM, Gornbein JA, Platt LD. Using administrative data to identify indications for elective primary cesarean delivery. *Health Services Research* 2002; 37:1387-1401.

Guise J, Berlin M, McDonough M, Osterweil P, Chan B, Helfand M. Safety of vaginal birth after cesarean: a systematic review. *Obstetrics & Gynecology* 2004; 103:420-429.

Harer WB Jr. Vaginal birth after cesarean delivery. *Journal of the American Medical Association* 2002; 287:2627-2630.

Hibbard JU, Ismail MA, Wang Y, Te C, Karrison T, Ismail MA. Failed vaginal birth after a cesarean section: How risky is it? I. Maternal morbidity. *American Journal of Obstetrics and Gynecology* 2001; 184:1365-1371.

Hook B, Kiwi R, Amini SB, Fanaroff A, Hack M. Neonatal morbidity after elective repeat cesarean section and trial of labor. *Pediatrics* 1997; 100:348-353.

Huang WH, Nakashima DK, Rumney PJ, Keegan KA Jr., Chan K. Interdelivery interval and the success of vaginal birth after cesarean delivery. *Obstetrics & Gynecology* 2002; 99:41-44.

Landon M. "The MFMU cesarean registry: risk of uterine rupture with a trial of labor in women with multiple and single prior cesarean delivery." Society for Maternal-Fetal Medicine annual meeting; February 2004.

Fisler RE, Cohen A, Ringer SA, Lieberman.E. Neoatal outcome after trial of labor compared with elective repeat cesarean section. *Birth* 2003; 30:83-88.

Lydon-Rochelle M, Holt VL, Easterling TR, Martin DP. Risk of uterine rupture during labor among women with a prior cesarean delivery. *New England Journal of Medicine* 2001; 345:3-8.

Mozurkewich EL, Hutton EK. Elective repeat cesarean delivery versus trial of labor: a meta-analysis of the literature from 1989 to 1999. *American Journal of Obstetrics and Gynecology* 2000; 183:1187-1197.

Odibo AO, Macones GA. Current concepts regarding vaginal birth after cesarean delivery. *Current Opinions in Obstetrics and Gynecology* 2003; 15:479-482.

Placek PJ, Taffel SM. Vaginal birth after cesarean (VBAC) in the 1980s. *American Journal of Public Health* 1988; 78:512-515.

Rucker MP, Rucker EM. A librarian looks at cesarean section. *Bulletin of the History of Medicine* 1951; 25:132-148.

Sewell JE. Cesarean section—a brief history. *American College of Obstetricians and Gynecologists*; 1993.

Shipp TD, Zelop CM, Cohen A, Repke JT, Lieberman E. Post-cesarean delivery fever and uterine rupture in a subsequent trial of labor. *Obstetrics & Gynecology* 2003; 101:136-139.

Shipp TD, Zelop C, Repke JU, Cohen A, Caughey AB, Liebeman E. The association of maternal age and symptomatic uterine rupture during a trial of labor after prior cesarean delivery. *Obstetrics & Gynecology* 2002; 99:585-588.

Shipp TD, Zelop CM, Repke JT, Cohen A, Lieberman E. Interdelivery interval and risk of symptomatic uterine rupture. *Obstetrics & Gynecology* 2001; 97:175-177.

Trolle F. *The History of Caesarean Section.* C.A. Reitzel Booksellers, Copenhagen: 1982.

Zelop CM, Shipp TD, Repke JT, Cohen A, Lieberman E. Outcomes of trial of labor following previous cesarean delivery among women with fetuses weighing >4000 g. *American Journal of Obstetrics and Gynecology* 2001; 185:903-905.

Resources

Where would we be without the Internet? There are a number of helpful Web sites dealing with childbirth, no matter whether you've scheduled a C-section or hope to avoid having one. Here are a few:

American College of Nurse-Midwives
Features a midwife locator.
http://www.acnm.org

American College of Obstetricians and Gynecologists
Order free copies of patient brochures about cesarean section, pain relief during labor and delivery, and other relevant subjects.
http://www.acog.org

Caesarean Birth
Launched by a mother who had two unplanned C-sections. Includes a chat room.
http://www.caesareanbirth.com

Doulas of North America (DONA)
Learn about the role of doulas and find help in locating one.
http://www.dona.com

International Cesarean Awareness Network (ICAN)
Formerly Cesarean Prevention Movement.
http://www.ican-online.org

Lamaze International
Features advice about reducing the chance of a cesarean delivery.
http://www.lamaze-childbirth.com

March of Dimes
Consumer information on a wide range of pregnancy and childbirth topics,
including c-sections.
www.marchofdimes.com

Maternity Center Association
New booklet, C-Section Myths/Reducing the Risks, can be downloaded
from the Web site.
http://www.maternitywise.org

MedlinePlus
A service of the U.S. National Library of Medicine and the National Institutes
of Health. Consumer information about c-sections.
http://www.nlm.nih.gov/medlineplus/cesareansection.html

National Association of Childbearing Centers (NACC)
FAQs on birth centers and birth center locator.
http://www.birthcenters.org

Vaginal Birth After Cesarean (VBAC)
Research-based information for mothers and health-care professionals.
http://www.vbac.com

INDEX